BALANCED

AND

BEAUTIFUL

KATRINA SCOTT

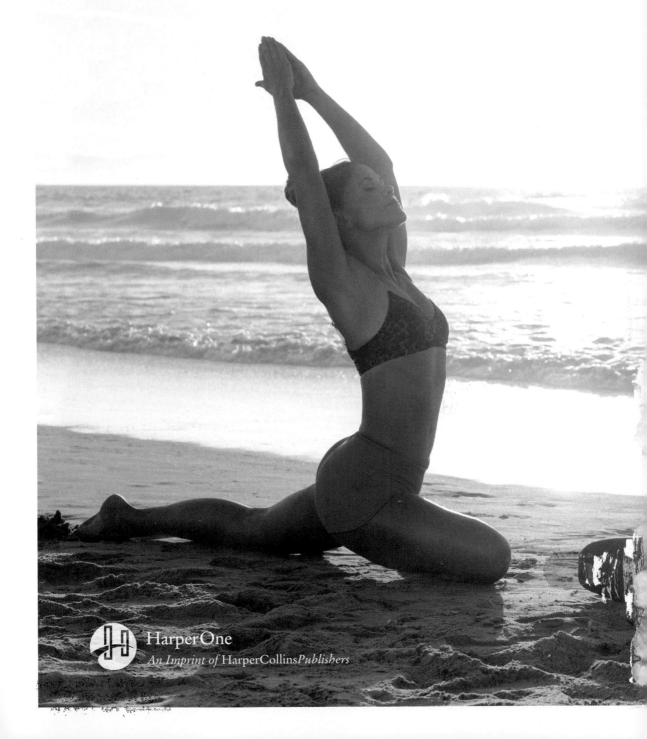

HarperOne
An Imprint of HarperCollinsPublishers

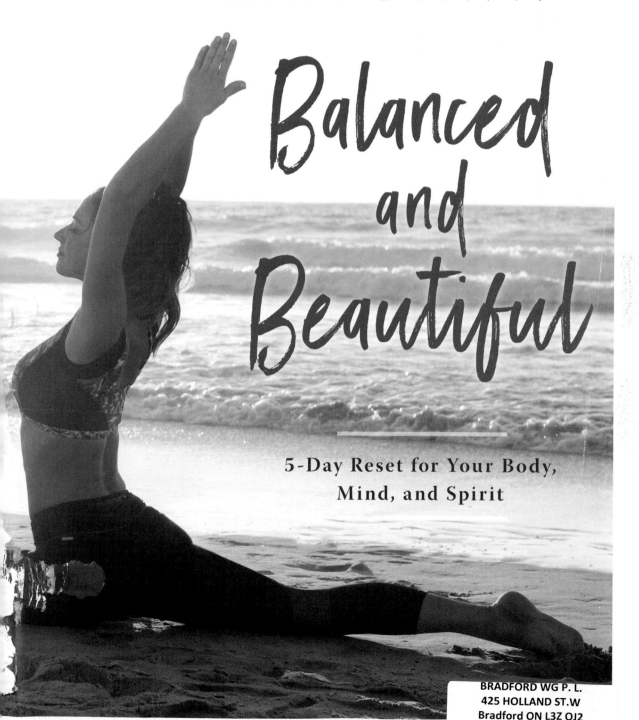

KARENA DAWN

Balanced and Beautiful

5-Day Reset for Your Body, Mind, and Spirit

HarperOne

Unless otherwise noted, all photographs courtesy of the authors.
Rolled towels image on page 40 courtesy didecs/Getty Images.
Lavender and essential oil bottles image on page 40 courtesy Amy_Lv/Getty Images.
Windows image on page 41 courtesy Mitshu/Getty Images.
Lavender, coffee, and notebook image on page 88 courtesy Julia_Sudnitskaya/Getty Images.
Water splash image on page 89 courtesy BlackJack3D/Getty Images.
Lipstick image on page 89 courtesy SergeyTay/Getty Images.
Lipstick smears image on page 183 courtesy Liliia Lysenko/Getty Images.
Candle image on page 228 courtesy PeopleImages/Getty Images.

This book contains advice and information relating to health care. It should be used to supplement rather than replace the advice of your doctor or another trained health professional. If you know or suspect you have a health problem, it is recommended that you seek your physician's advice before embarking on any medical program or treatment. All efforts have been made to ensure the accuracy of the information contained in this book as of the date of publication. This publisher and the authors disclaim liability for any medical outcomes that may occur as a result of applying the methods suggested in this book.

HarperCollins books may be purchased for educational, business, or sales promotional use. For information, please email the Special Markets Department at SPsales@harpercollins.com.

FIRST EDITION

Designed by Janet Evans-Scanlon

Library of Congress Cataloging-in-Publication Data has been applied for.

ISBN 978-0-06-284348-7
ISBN 978-0-06-287748-2 (Target)

18 19 20 21 22   LSC   10 9 8 7 6 5 4 3 2 1

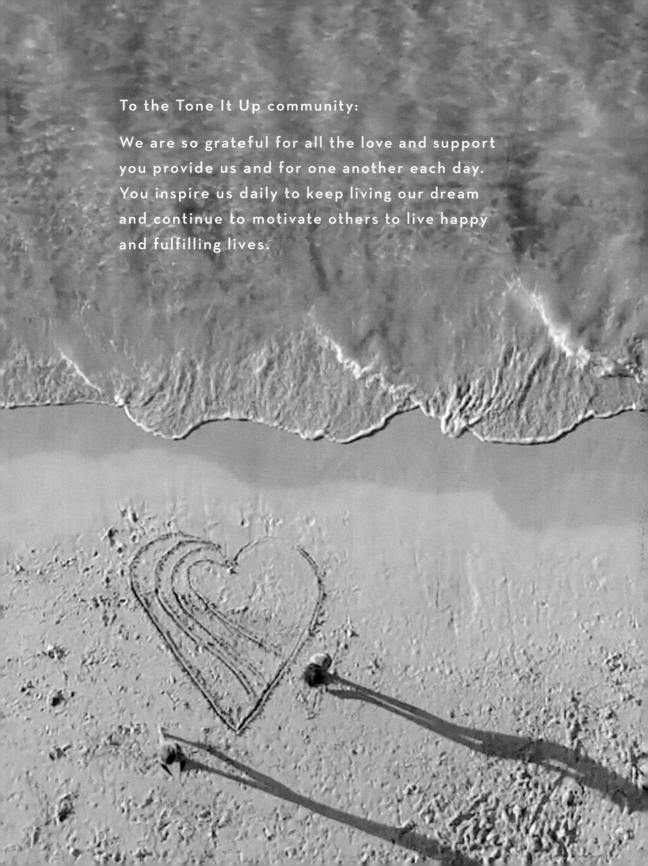

To the Tone It Up community:

We are so grateful for all the love and support you provide us and for one another each day. You inspire us daily to keep living our dream and continue to motivate others to live happy and fulfilling lives.

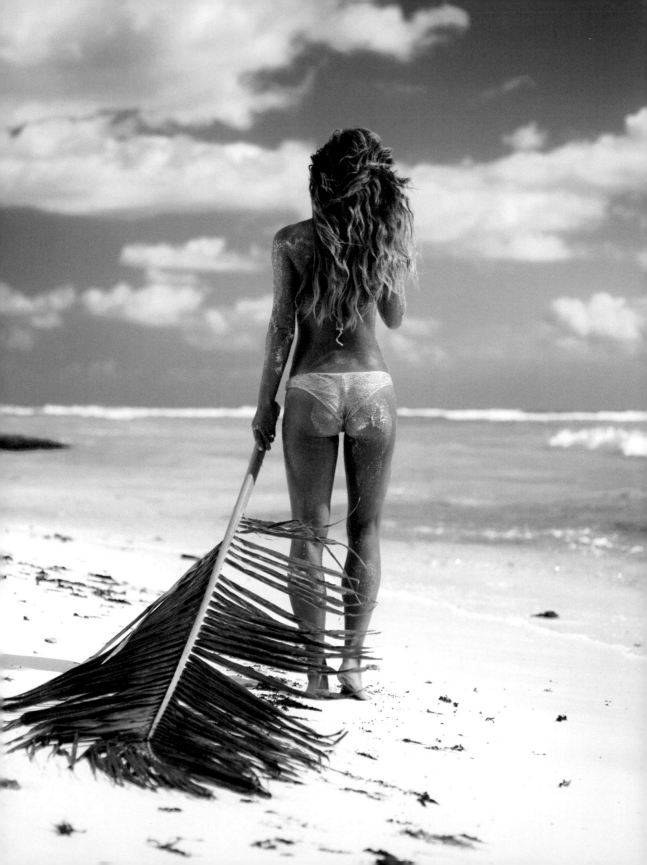

CONTENTS

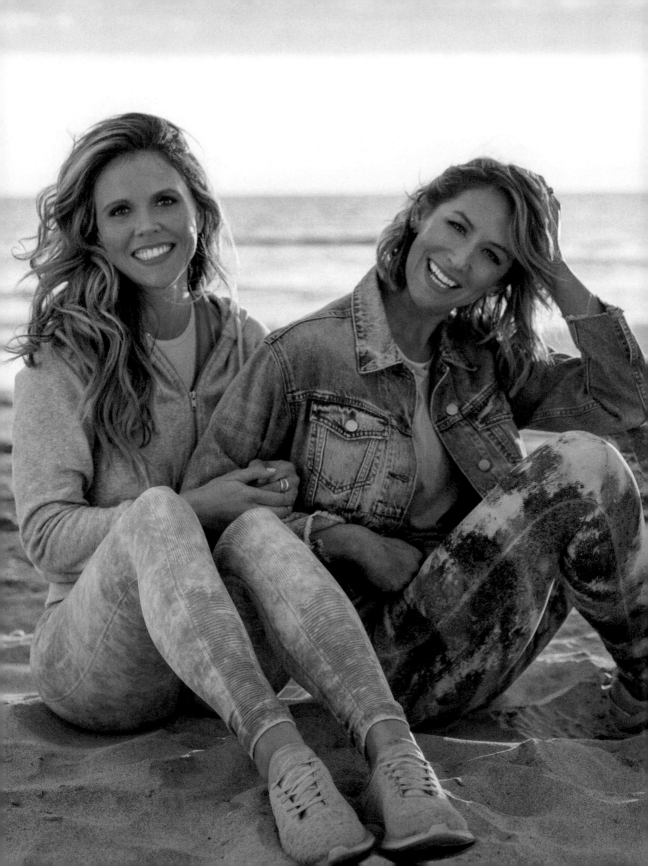

Hey, Gorgeous!

We're so excited you're here. Just by opening this book, you've done something incredible for *you*. Congratulations on taking that first step to better yourself and begin your journey of passion, purpose, and self-love. Throughout these pages, you'll feel empowered, uplifted, connected, and, of course, balanced and beautiful—because that's what the Tone It Up lifestyle is all about.

If you're new to Tone It Up, welcome! Here you'll find a loving community of women who support and empower one another to live their healthiest and most confident lives. We're Karena and Katrina, best friends and your fitness and lifestyle coaches. We created Tone It Up to make sure every woman feels her very best and achieves all her dreams—because they are possible, and the best *you* is possible.

As women, we so often put others first. We're nurturers and we want to care for everyone around us—but when we take time to prioritize ourselves, we are better partners, parents, girlfriends, wives, and leaders. Through the amazing journey of creating Tone It Up, we realized that life is truly about infusing mindfulness into everything we do.

It's about finding balance not just within us but also within everyone in our lives.

We've dedicated ourselves to connecting women to one another and to being a part of their journeys. *You* have so much to say, so much to give, so much wisdom and heart to share. It's your knowledge that helped us create this book for you.

Balanced and Beautiful is about so much more than fitness. It's about aligning yourself with positivity each day and awakening your most beautiful and authentic self.

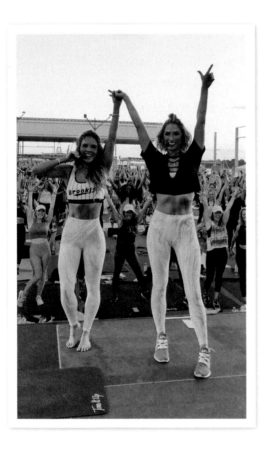

We totally understand too how life can fall out of balance. For whatever reason—a challenging life transition, an unexpected health issue, a stressful month with work, conflicts—sometimes you get thrown off your game, and this can create a ripple effect that touches every aspect of your life. We're going to show you how to look at every obstacle as a lesson, every closed door as an opportunity, and how to balance your life, ensuring that you always feel an abundance of love and support.

We drew a lot of inspiration for this book from our first-ever Tone It Up Tour in 2017. Going on tour was a longtime dream for us, and we hit the road to visit fifteen cities in thirty days. Women came from all over the world (we even met some who flew in from

Sri Lanka, Dubai, and Romania!) to work out, to fuel their souls with inspiration, and to connect with the community.

In every city, we hosted meet and greets, which we love because they give us the opportunity to connect with women one-on-one. Through hugs, smiles, tears, and rosé, we got to hear so many stories of strength, perseverance, friendship, community, and love. Women told us about how they met their best friends through the Tone It Up community, how they lost over 50 pounds, how they've been through tough times, moved across the country, faced heartaches, miscarriages, breakups, divorces, cancer, and how they found the courage to shift professional careers to chase their dreams. One thing stayed consistent: they all felt supported and brave enough to face their challenges head-on because they have the Tone It Up community. Hearing this over and over meant more to us than anything ever before.

We had moments when we looked at each other in awe and were just totally blown away by these women. We felt unbelievably honored and humbled to be trusted with so many of their personal experiences and to play even a small part in their journeys.

That's the power of community! The power of women who support, encourage, and inspire one another. Which is why we want to bring the joy of Tone It Up to every woman. We always say our mission is to make the world a better place and to bring more positivity into every woman's life.

This book you hold in your hands is for *you*. It will explore how to take care of you—no matter who you are or what you're going through. Like a best girlfriend, it will always be here to offer insight and love. With every turn of the page, you will feel refreshed, motivated, inspired, energized, relaxed, and ready to live your most balanced and beautiful life.

How It All Began

Let's back up a little so we can tell you how this beautiful journey started. It was a Friday night at the gym, and we were both new to Manhattan Beach, California. Neither of us knew anyone in town, so it was the perfect time for both of us to meet a new girlfriend. I—Katrina—was working as a personal trainer, and I noticed that Karena always came in to read and work out on the exercise bike. One night, I introduced myself. I went right up to her while she was stretching and said, "My, you're flexible. Do you do yoga?" We still joke about my "pickup line"!

That led to our first yoga date, and then we started going for long walks with coffee or smoothies. As we got to know each other, we realized that we both shared the same passion and vision. Fitness positively affected our lives, and we both wanted it to touch the lives of women around the world. We talked endlessly about creating a community that connected women so they could find support through girlfriends, just like we did, and live their best lives through health and fitness.

So with just the two of us, a video camera on a tripod, and determination in hand, Tone It Up was born! We recorded cooking segments and workout videos on the beach and posted them on ToneItUp.com. We learned so much—how to use lighting, video editing, and sound equipment. Over time, we learned about each other's backstories and discovered that we both had deeper reasons for our passion for fitness than simply wanting to be in shape. Knowing that this lifestyle was just as much an emotional journey as a physical one helped us stay focused on our goals and remain clear on our mission for women.

We want to share our stories with you, not only so you get to know us better but also as inspiration for you on your own journey—what has brought you to this very moment in your beautiful life!

Get to Know Us

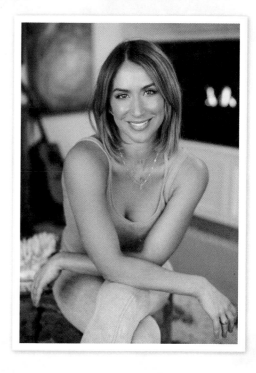

KARENA'S STORY

I fell in love with sports and fitness while growing up in Indiana. I did my first half marathon with my dad when I was only twelve years old, and I watched my mom doing Jane Fonda and Kathy Smith home workouts on VHS. I remember, for one of my first school projects, I created a workout video in my living room. When my life became complicated and challenging during my teenage years—my mom was diagnosed with a serious mental illness—I was devastated, turned inward, and found myself self-destructing, eating poorly, and treating my body horribly. I started taking drugs as an escape from the confusion, anger, and depression I was struggling with. I didn't believe in myself or have the confidence to actually *live* my life.

I eventually reached a breaking point, and I had to choose a path. One road would lead me to a worsening addiction and a shaky future with few options. The other would lead me out into the light, where I could find the strength to overcome my painful past, make the changes

I knew I had to make so *I* would control my life instead of *it* controlling *me*, and find my purpose. I knew I was smart and could make something wonderful happen. I also knew I deserved better than the low expectations I'd set for myself. First and foremost, I knew I needed to rediscover a love for myself, because everything starts with love.

So I chose the right road, and immediately made a crazy decision: to do my first triathlon! I'd always loved running and competing in races when I was younger, and I figured the intense training I'd need to do would keep my thoughts and behavior from straying back into harmful patterns. And I was right! Of course, on race day I was a quivering bundle of nerves, but *I did it*. I kept going even when my muscles screamed at me to stop and my brain told me to just give in and sit down. I pushed past that negativity and crossed that finish line with tears of joy in my eyes. In that moment, my life totally changed. I realized I had the power within me to accomplish anything I committed to.

I ran more and more triathlons, started doing yoga and meditation, got certified as a personal trainer and nutrition coach, then went on to get my yoga teacher certification. I began working as a sports and fitness model and an on-camera spokesperson for major athletic brands, appearing on the covers of *Triathlete* and other magazines, like *Runner's World, Shape, Women's Health*, and *Self*. I looked at my accomplishments and felt so grateful for the amazing journey I'd been on and how far I'd gone, thanks to determination, hard work, and an unwavering belief in using the power of positivity and visualization to reach my goals.

And then I met my best friend, Kat, and life was never the same again. We combined our dreams and our passion to create something even more beautiful!

KATRINA'S STORY

My fitness journey started at a young age, and it shaped my entire life. When I was in elementary school, I was the heaviest girl in class. Like a lot of kids, I was teased. I'll never forget going to the mall with my mom when I was eleven. We went into a trendy store where all the girls in my class shopped. The woman at the front stopped my mom on the way in and said, "Ma'am, I don't think we have anything here that will fit your daughter." I pretended not to hear, but I was crushed. Not because I was heavy, but because my mom was facing what I faced every day in school. I remember crying myself to sleep that night, into my pillow. I wanted to wear what other girls my age were wearing—I wanted to feel healthy and confident. Later that month, I went to my parents and asked for help. They were always so supportive—not once had they ever told me I needed to lose weight. My dad wanted to make me happy, so he went into action, transforming our basement into a home gym, fully equipped with weights, a bench, a treadmill, mirrors, and music. I would come home from school and blast music, run, work out, and dream about being a healthier, happier me. This is when I started creating workouts and meal plans from what I was learning from fitness and nutrition magazines and books.

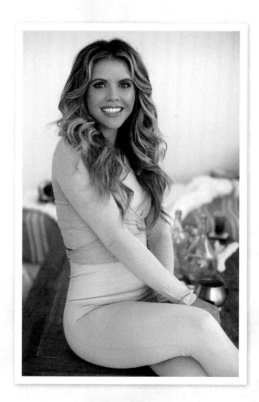

When I was old enough to drive, I got a job at a vitamin store. Learning all about nutrients inspired me to go to school for health science and exercise physiology.

The first certification I received was for group fitness. I remember nervously preparing a playlist for my first class on campus, wondering if anyone would show up. As I turned the corner into the workout room with my headset and playlist, I saw more than fifty girls in line to take the class, including my supportive roommates! I was shaking. From that moment on, I fell in love with the energy of teaching workout classes. It meant the world to me to see all the girls pile in after school and do something for themselves. It was a place for girls to come together, chat before class, and empower one another to feel amazing. After class, I would watch everyone leave together, having just met,

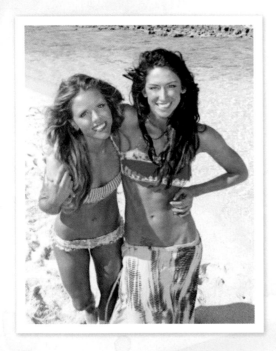

and I knew it was so much more than an abs and booty class—it was creating friendships. After earning my bachelor's degree in health science and fitness, I worked as a master trainer in Boston and started creating fitness videos on YouTube. Completely awestruck by the millions of views of my videos, I knew I could make an impact on fitness for women. So with big dreams of doing fitness on the beach, I moved to California. Then serendipity brought Karena and me together—which was the beginning of something beautiful and life changing for us and our soon-to-be community: the TIU team!

Welcome to Tone It Up!

Since that fateful day we met in the gym, we're proud to say that Tone It Up has grown into a worldwide community of millions of strong, beautiful women. On ToneItUp.com and through your Studio Tone It Up app, you'll find daily workouts, lifestyle challenges, and fitness classes you can take live with the community. On the website, you can also find our Tone It Up Protein, which we use in many of the recipes in this book. The coolest part about the app is that you can invite girlfriends to take the class with you—no matter where they live! You can chat before and after class in the studio and hold each other accountable. There's magic in knowing that you're not alone on this journey.

We also offer an endless supply of science-backed fitness and nutrition advice. Our Tone It Up Nutrition Plan includes meal-by-meal guides, grocery lists, what to eat each day, thousands of delicious recipes, and special meal plans you can use for events, vacation, or big life changes like a wedding, college, a growing family, and so much more!

Your Guide to Feeling Balanced and Beautiful

In this book, you'll find 5 chapters representing the 5-day reset journey: "Refresh," "Motivate," "Inspire," "Energize," and "Relax"—the perfect combination for your most balanced and beautiful life.

Each day of this journey includes everything you need: Girl Talk (we all need girlfriend advice every now and then), a Spiritual Guide (to emotionally connect with the most important person in your life—*you*), a Workout Guide (to leave you feeling strong), a Recipe Guide (to nourish your body with the most delicious recipes), a Girlfriend Guide (to give you the tools to live your most fulfilled life with strong friendships), an Action Guide (to put your new power into play), and a place to Connect with the Tone It Up Community (for stories and advice from others).

You'll also find mantras to brighten your day and plenty of inspiring quotes in the Vision Board sections. You'll use meditation to center yourself in the mornings, follow our Beauty Tips to feel gorgeous, and a list of some of our favorite books to curl up with when you need to unwind after a long day. Want to throw a fabulous girls' night? We share our top ideas to make lasting memories with your friends. Plus, at the end of every chapter, a section called Reflect encourages you to write down your thoughts about each day's focus. By the end of these five days, you'll feel so empowered you'll want to keep going. And any time you feel the need for a refresh, pick up this book to feel balanced and beautiful.

What if we told you that you were already *balanced and beautiful*? What if we told you that all your strengths are already within the depths of your heart? You already have the foundation and the drive. A breakthrough occurs when you realize that what you've been looking for has been within your reach all along. We're not here to tell you to be inspired, to feel motivated, or to find balance; we're here to be your mirror, to show you that you already embody all of those attributes.

Visualize who you want to be—your most beautiful, grounded, and authentic self. Who is she? From this moment moving forward, we want you to take every action, every single day, to emulate her. Every decision you make, every move you make, and every word you speak is with the intent to be her. Soon enough, you will radiate all the beauty you imagine and empower the women around you to do the same for themselves—and that right there is *powerful*.

Are you ready for this?

Yes! We know you are!

TAKE A MOMENT, CLOSE YOUR EYES, AND IMAGINE YOURSELF...

- You're *refreshed*, taking on everything you set your heart to.

- You're *motivated* to accomplish your goals and chase your dreams.

- You're *inspired* and empowering everyone around you.

- You're *energized*, ready to challenge yourself in new ways.

- You're *relaxed*, enjoying time with loved ones.

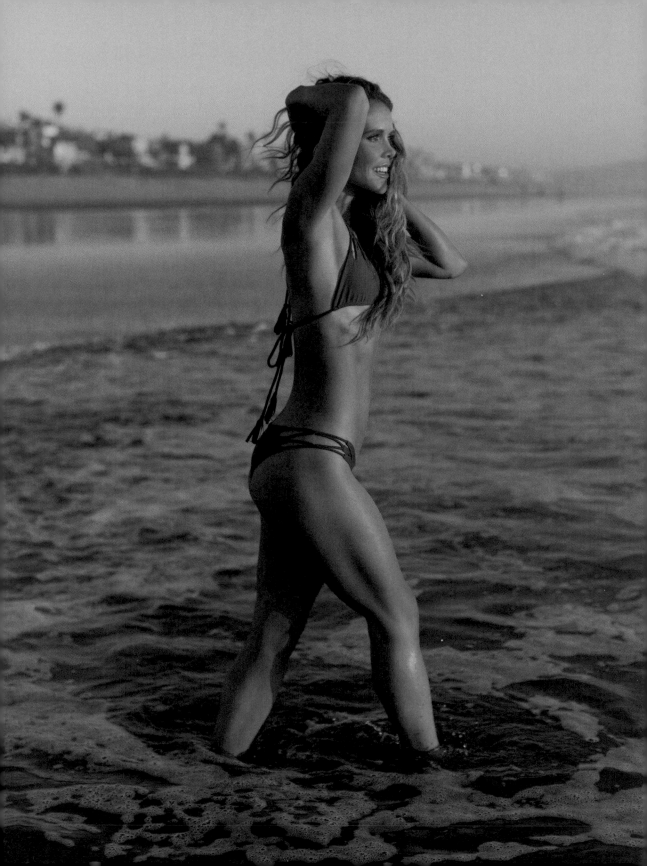

1

Refresh

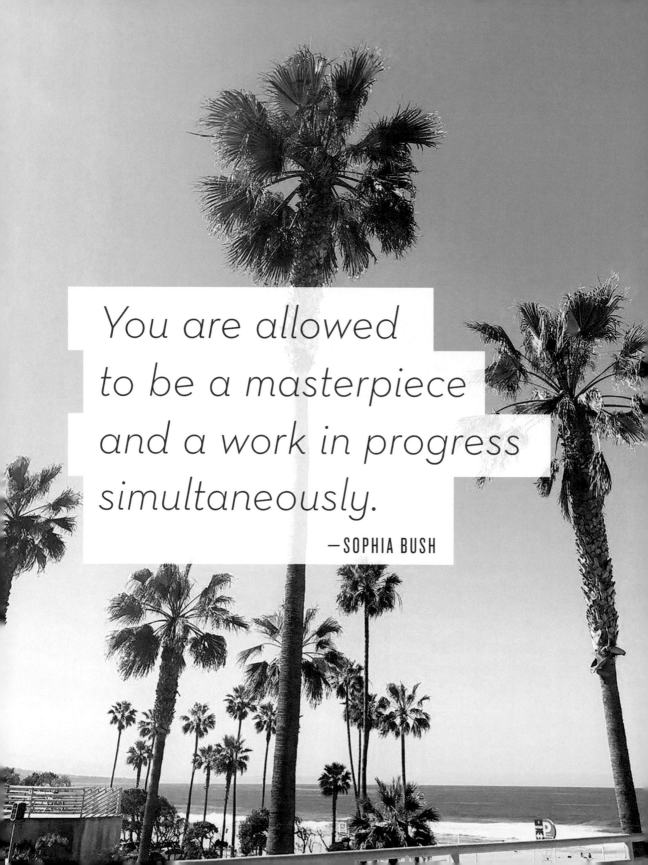

You are allowed
to be a masterpiece
and a work in progress
simultaneously.

—SOPHIA BUSH

GIRL TALK
to Refresh

KATRINA When I just thought of the word "refresh," the first thing that came to mind was pressing REFRESH on my browser. Funny, because that's probably what we all need a refresh from! So let's do the same thing to our lives. This chapter, "Refresh," is something you can come back to as many times as you want. Once you've completed your five days in this book, you can press REFRESH again! Life is about re-creating ourselves, setting new goals, sometimes falling off a path, and then starting over again—with more strength and perseverance than ever before.

A few months ago, Karena and I needed a refresh. We were working so much, even through weekends for months on end, and we forgot to take a moment to pause, breathe, and reflect. So we set everything aside and planned a full day of just setting up our lives for balance and success. In the morning, we went for a long walk and talked about our goals and how we would achieve them. We recognized our strengths and weaknesses and talked about how we would overcome our obstacles. We then took a sixty-minute yoga sculpt class, which uses weights for a total-body workout. Afterward, we felt like we had sweat out the last two months of pent-up stress and deadlines. We came out feeling lighter, cleansed, and at peace. From there, we created a detox meal plan and prepped meals for the next five days. We felt inspired and motivated to take on the next challenge and get back to work.

So whenever you feel like you're lacking motivation or inspiration, start with a refresh. You'll be able to dive into the next chapter of your life with so much more energy!

refresh

SPIRITUAL GUIDE
to Refresh

KARENA Essential oils are my absolute favorite. They make me feel so refreshed. I grew up in a home where incense and candles were constantly burning, so aromatherapy has always been a part of my life. I've found that scents can lift your mood and give you energy. They can also be the perfect refresher and rejuvenator at the end of the day. When I'm in the shower, I like to dab oil on my wrists, rub them together, and inhale. I also stash oils on my bedside table, throughout my house, in my purse, and in the drawer next to my desk at HQ so they're always on hand.

One of the best ways to take advantage of essential oils is with an oil diffuser. Letting the scents gently fill the air will instantly refresh your environment. Choose any of the oils I've listed next, and have fun experimenting with combinations. You only need to put a few drops in a diffuser for each use, so a little bottle of an essential oil will last a long time.

What Refreshes Me

I'm refreshed by a good night's sleep, fresh fruit, a morning of mindfulness and gratitude, and then, of course, getting physical!

Karena

What Refreshes Me

I feel the most refreshed when I get to work out in the fresh air outside. I also feel refreshed after I shower and journal my intentions for the day. Oh . . . and taking a bra off at the end of the day! Wow, what a feeling.

Katrina

Basil. One of the best essential oils for relieving tension, basil is also the ideal choice if you want to create a refreshing massage oil. It works best mixed with a neutral carrier oil like jojoba or sweet almond.

Bergamot. This citrus oil relieves stress and anxiety, is purifying, and creates balance in your mood.

Geranium. This essential oil is extra refreshing when you put it in a diffuser. It's sort of sweet and spicy at the same time, and I always feel the stress melting away when the scent permeates the room.

Lavender. One of the best-known scents for refreshing (and relaxing), lavender is the oil I always use to unwind before bed. Research has shown that lavender improves sleep quality, decreases stress and anxiety, and quiets your mind before you drift off.

Lemon. Lemon oil—and any of the other citrus oils, like lime or wild orange—will instantly cleanse and purify the air, and it always uplifts my spirits.

Lemongrass. This is another oil known for its refreshing properties. It smells deliciously lemony.

Rosemary. I love this oil mixed with bath salts for a detoxifying soak in my tub. It's also excellent for clarity.

Ylang-ylang. This essential oil smells so good and is one of my go-tos when my mood needs a boost—it's refreshing and balancing at the same time.

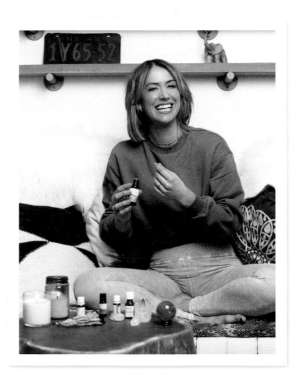

refresh

WORKOUT GUIDE
to Refresh

We all want to feel like we're light on our toes and our heart is shining forward. There's nothing worse than feeling the opposite: sluggish and tired. When we get into a rut or a week of work when we don't have time for exercise, let alone a moment to dry our hair or make a meal, we need to take a step back and refresh. After talking with entrepreneurs, busy boss babes, students, and moms in the community, we've come to realize that we're all in the same boat. We just want to be able to take time for ourselves and to feel confident and healthy.

A workout gives you a feeling like all the built-up energy that's been sitting inside you is finally out. When you move, you feel a release of tension. After completing yoga, boxing, HIIT (high-intensity interval training), dance, or a Studio Tone It Up workout, you will feel so refreshed that you will kind of forget what you felt like before.

The best way to refresh the entire body is to work the *entire body*. Using every muscle boosts your metabolism, uses stored sugars in your muscles, and sculpts you from head to toe.

Exercises to Refresh Your Whole Body

To get the most out of this workout, or any workout with weights, start with a heavier set of weights (12 to 15 pounds) and complete as many reps as you can with proper form, then drop down to a lower weight. This is called a "drop set." It helps you get stronger, form lean muscle, and sculpt that gorgeous tush!

Do *three circuits* of the following exercises on each side of your body:

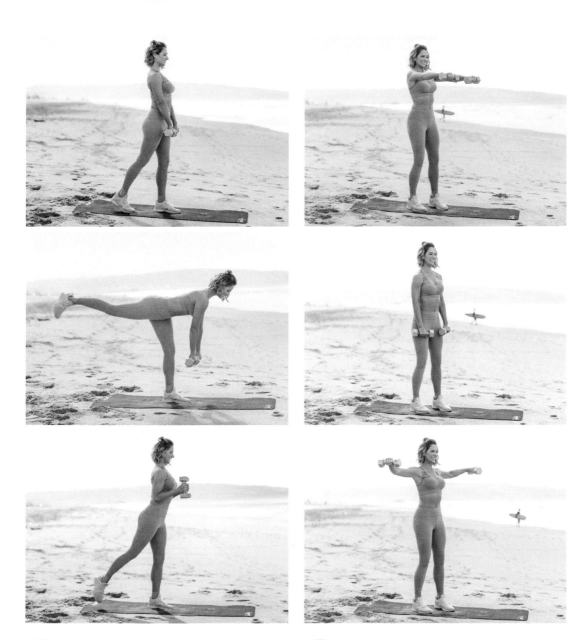

1 *Single Leg Dead Lift with Hammer Curl*

15 REPS ON EACH SIDE

2 *Forward and Lateral Raises*

10 REPS OF EACH, 20 REPS TOTAL

refresh

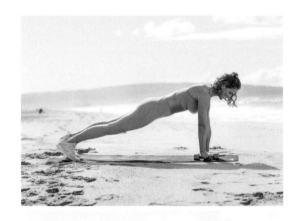

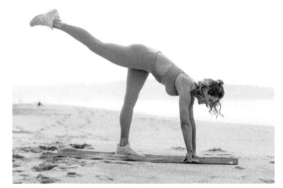

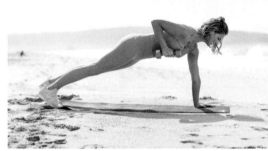

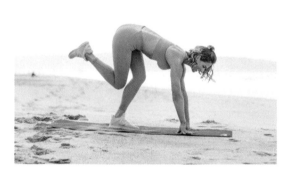

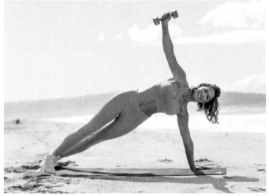

3 *Forward Fold*
Curtsy Squat

15 REPS ON EACH SIDE

4 *Plank Row to Press*

15 REPS ON EACH SIDE

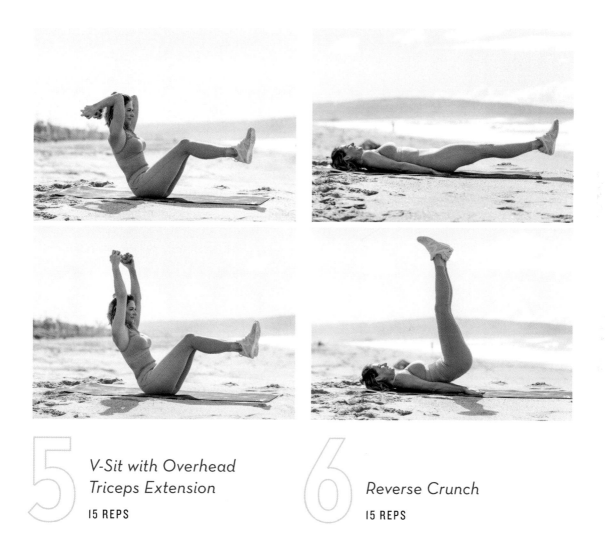

5   *V-Sit with Overhead Triceps Extension*
15 REPS

6   *Reverse Crunch*
15 REPS

refresh

RECIPE GUIDE
to Refresh

Imagine iced tea on a hot summer day, fresh lemon water when you wake up, and a refreshing smoothie after a tough workout. Food can really make you feel some kinda way! We put together a few of our favorite refreshing recipes that will leave you feeling invigorated.

MORNING MOCKTAIL

Serves 1

We created this recipe the day we made our detox plan. It's our go-to in the morning. It hydrates you while balancing your alkalinity and boosting your metabolism. An all-around perfect way to kick off your day!

8 ounces water
Juice of ½ lemon

1 tablespoon apple cider vinegar
Pinch of ground cayenne (optional)

In a glass, stir to combine all the ingredients, and enjoy!

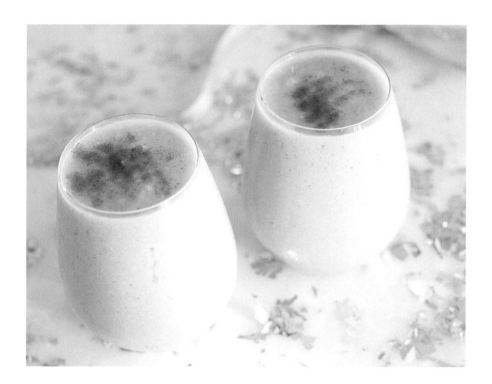

K&K CLEANSE SMOOTHIE

Serves 1

Name a more refreshing smoothie . . . we'll wait. Seriously, this one takes the *kale*!

1 cup coconut water

1 scoop vanilla Tone It Up Protein

¼ cup spinach

¼ cup kale

½ cup frozen chopped mango

1 tablespoon ground flaxseeds

½-inch piece fresh ginger, peeled

Pinch of ground cayenne (optional)

In a high-speed blender, blend all the ingredients until the mixture is smooth, and enjoy!

refresh

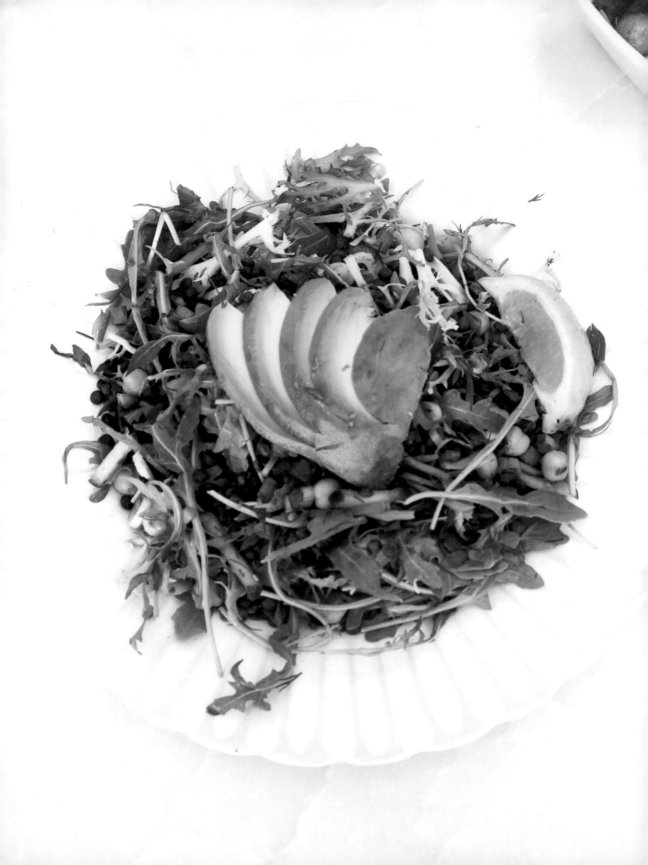

AVOCADO LENTIL SALAD
with LEMON DIJON DRESSING

Serves 1 (with enough dressing for 4 salads)

Probably our favorite lunch—ever.

FOR THE SALAD

¼ cup cooked brown lentils

1 carrot, shredded

¼ cup chopped radish

¼ cup chopped fennel bulb

2 cups arugula

2 tablespoons garbanzo beans

1 tablespoon unsalted sunflower seeds, shelled

¼ avocado, peeled, pitted, and sliced

1 lemon slice

FOR THE DRESSING

1 tablespoon diced shallot

2 teaspoons Dijon mustard

1 teaspoon honey

2 tablespoons olive oil

1 tablespoon red wine vinegar

Juice of 1 lemon

In a bowl, toss together the lentils, carrot, radish, fennel, arugula, beans, and sunflower seeds, then set the salad aside.

Combine all the ingredients for the dressing in a food processor, and pulse until the mixture is well combined.

Toss the salad with 1 tablespoon of the dressing, garnish with the slices of avocado, then dress the salad with an extra squeeze of the lemon slice.

The remaining dressing can keep for up to a week in the fridge (you'll need some for Day 5's menu).

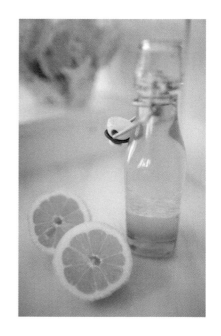

refresh

SLIMMING SOUP

Serves 4

This metabolism-boosting, liver-cleansing, slimming soup is perfect for any meal. Having this as your lunch, with a side salad, or as an afternoon pick-me-up will leave you feeling so refreshed.

1 teaspoon olive oil

1 yellow onion, diced

3 cups diced carrots

1 cup red lentils

1-inch piece fresh ginger, peeled and diced

1 teaspoon ground cumin

1/2 teaspoon ground coriander

1/8 teaspoon ground cayenne

Pinch of salt

4 cups vegetable broth

In a large pot set over medium heat, warm the olive oil, then add the onion and sauté it for 3 to 5 minutes.

Add to the pot the carrots, lentils, ginger, cumin, coriander, cayenne, salt, and broth. Bring the mixture to a boil, then reduce the heat and cover the pot. Simmer the soup for 20 minutes.

Carefully pour the soup into a blender and blend it on a low setting until it's smooth, or use an immersion blender while it's still in the pot.

The soup can be saved in glass containers in the fridge for up to five days.

BEET THE BLOAT SALAD

Serves 2

1 cup shredded beet

1 cup shredded carrot

1 apple, cored and diced

¼ cup unsalted
sunflower seeds

Juice of 1 lemon

2 tablespoons olive oil

Pinch of salt

Toss all the ingredients together in a bowl, and enjoy!

REFRESHING SPRITZERS

Add these refreshing combos to sparkling water.
We also love adding ice cubes with edible flowers
such as violets, rose petals, or nasturtiums in them.
Cheers!

Raspberries and
lime juice

Strawberries and
lemon juice

Watermelon chunks
and mint leaves

Crushed apples and
ground cinnamon

Coconut water and
lime juice

Pomegranate seeds
and lemon juice

refresh

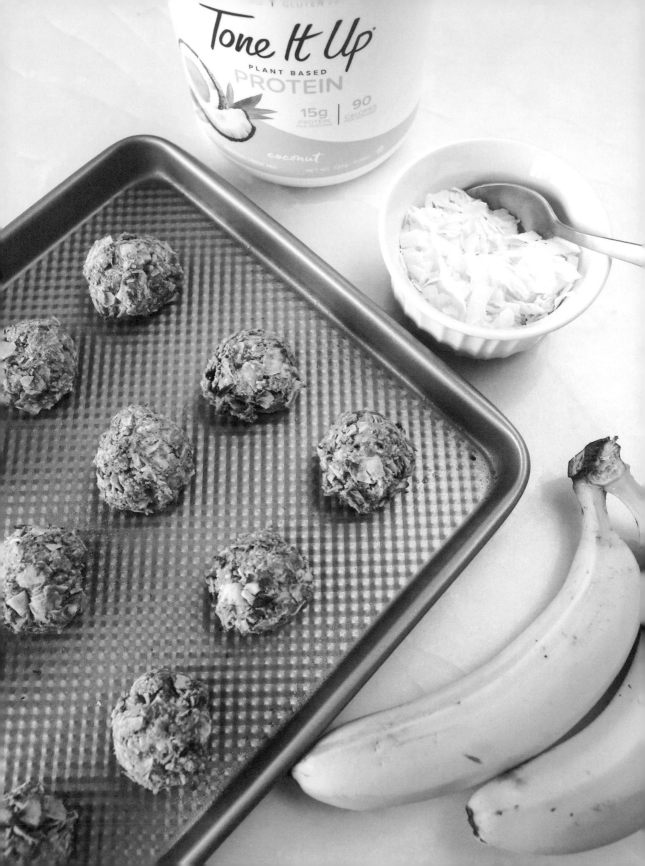

COCONUTTY MACAROONS

Makes 14

2 bananas, mashed

1 egg or flax egg,
lightly whisked

1 cup unsweetened
coconut flakes

2 scoops vanilla
Tone It Up Protein

Coconut oil spray

Preheat the oven to 350°F.

In a bowl, stir together the bananas, egg, coconut flakes, and Tone It Up Protein until the mixture is well combined.

Coat a cookie sheet with the coconut oil spray, then spoon the mixture onto the sheet to make 14 macaroons.

Bake the macaroons for 13 minutes, or until they are firm.

refresh

DETOXIFYING
FOODS AND SIPS

Sometimes we too need a refresh. We love doing the detox meal plan every now and then, which includes everything listed here. Download your complimentary meal plan at ToneItUp.com.

For detoxifying effects on a regular basis, incorporate these superpowers:

- Milk thistle and dandelion root are *healing teas* known to help the liver. Drink a warm cup of either tea to feel the benefits. (Consult your doctor if you're breastfeeding.)

- *Chlorophyll* is not so borophyll! Dark leafy greens are packed with nutrients to make you glow. Their chlorophyll helps the body get rid of environmental toxins and heavy metals, and they're packed with vitamins and antioxidants to fight inflammation.

- Care for some turmeric? First, add freshly ground black pepper! *Turmeric* is a bright orange spice containing an active compound called curcumin, which is an anti-inflammatory powerhouse. Whenever you use turmeric, add a dash of black pepper too. A compound in black pepper called piperine helps increase absorption of curcumin in your body by up to 2,000 percent!

- *Berries* are one of nature's superfoods—they're packed with antioxidants. We often enjoy a morning smoothie with blueberries, almond milk, frozen bananas or cauliflower rice, and vanilla Tone It Up Protein.

- We've always loved *apple cider vinegar*. We have a shot of it every morning. It not only detoxifies your body but helps boost your metabolism. See page 10 for how to make a morning "mocktail" with ACV. Talk about refreshing! ACV is also amazing on salads and in dressings.

- *Asparagus* helps detoxify the liver and also naturally banishes bloat. Beach, please!

- When life gives you lemons . . . make *lemonade*. Lemons stimulate the liver, and their natural citric acid helps your digestion. Add fresh lemon juice and crushed strawberries to sparkling water for a healthy sparkling pink lemonade.

- Drink up, babe! The key to feeling refreshed is hydration. *Water* carries nutrients to your cells and helps the kidneys flush toxins from your body. Lots of water is needed for all your organs to carry out their duties, so aim to drink at least half your body weight in ounces of H_2O a day. For a more flavorful (and detoxifying) sip, add a little squeeze of lemon to your water.

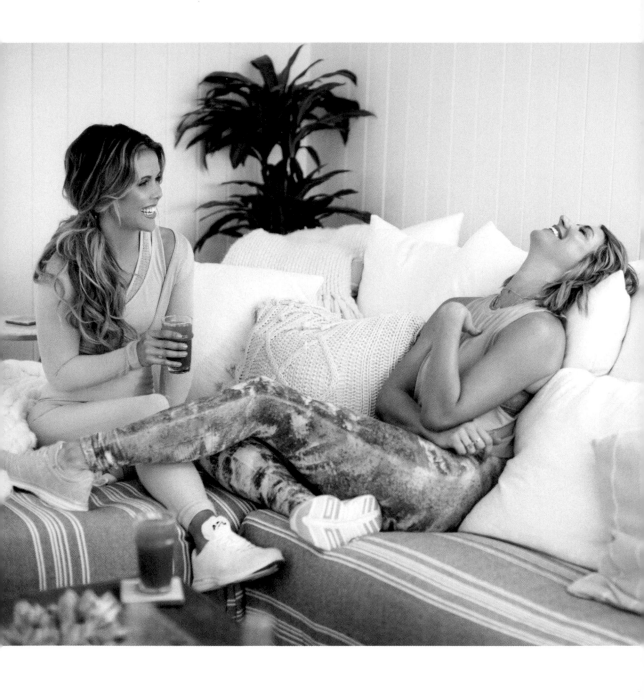

GIRLFRIEND GUIDE
to Refresh

Spa Night In

KARENA Every girl needs a little night of beauty. One of our favorite things to do is host our girlfriends for a Spa Night In. Kat and I will make healthy food, serve our refreshing spritzers (page 15), and pamper ourselves—face and eye masks, nails, hair, the whole works! We love to make our own face masks. They're as much fun to make with your friends as they are to use.

Grab a bunch of jars to store the masks in, so you can send any extra home with your girls. (Double or triple the following recipes, depending on how many babes you got.)

BUT FIRST . . . COFFEE

Rub this mask all over your hot bod—we're not kidding! A coffee scrub will help increase circulation, exfoliate your skin, and reduce the appearance of cellulite. I'm in!

1 ½ cups coarsely ground coffee

½ cup raw sugar or sea salt

3 tablespoons coconut oil, melted, or olive oil

In a bowl, combine the ground coffee with the sugar or sea salt.

Add the coconut or olive oil, and mix until it becomes a thick paste. Add more oil as needed to achieve your desired consistency.

After a warm shower or bath, apply the mask to your skin, making sure to rub it all over your legs, booty, and midsection. Use firm, circular motions, and if desired, let it sit for a few minutes before rinsing it off with warm water. Remember to use a fine-mesh drain strainer in your tub to prevent the grounds from causing any plumbing problems!

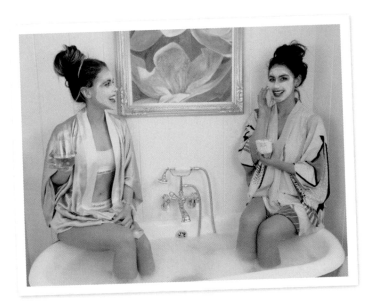

AVO-MOISTURIZING MASK

This mask is super hydrating and totally edible—great for Taco Tuesdays! The natural oils in avocado help hydrate your face and plump up any dry areas. The yogurt provides riboflavin, vitamins B_6 and B_{12}, and calcium, and its lactic acid helps smooth skin and tighten pores. Honey is naturally antibacterial, so it's great for acne and breakouts. Olé!

1/2 ripe avocado, peeled and pitted	1 teaspoon yogurt 1 teaspoon honey

In a bowl, combine all the ingredients until the mixture is a smooth consistency.

Apply it to your face evenly, and let it sit for 10 to 15 minutes.

Rinse the mask off with warm water, a face wash, and a washcloth.

SUGAR . . . OH, HONEY, HONEY

Oats have antioxidant and anti-inflammatory powers to moisturize and heal skin. This mask is great if your skin is dry and itchy. The honey and sugar scrub will make you glow fo-dayzzzz!

1/2 cup yogurt 1/3 cup organic oat flour (or oats ground into oat flour)	2 teaspoons honey 1 teaspoon sugar

In a bowl, combine all the ingredients.

Apply just enough of the mask to completely cover your face except your eyes, nose, and mouth. Let it sit for 10 to 20 minutes.

Rinse the mask off with warm water, a face wash, and a washcloth.

refresh

CITRUS GLOW

This mask will instantly brighten dull skin thanks to vitamins B_6 and C in the bananas and the soothing power of the honey. The citric acid in oranges is a natural alpha hydroxy acid, which exfoliates and cleans your skin. Way cheaper than going to get a chemical peel!

½ banana, mashed

1 tablespoon freshly squeezed orange juice

1 tablespoon coconut oil, melted

In a bowl, combine all the ingredients.

Apply the mixture to your face, and let it sit for 10 to 15 minutes.

Rinse the mask off with lukewarm water, and moisturize.

PLUMP AND PUMP ME UP

Pumpkin is packed with fruit enzymes and alpha hydroxy acids, which help renew skin cells. This will brighten and smooth your face. Pumpkin also contains antioxidant vitamins A and C to help boost collagen production—yes, please! The egg white will help tighten pores with its astringent properties, and the lemon is antibacterial, helping prevent breakouts.

¼ cup pumpkin puree

1 egg

2 teaspoons honey

Tiny splash of freshly squeezed lemon juice

In a bowl, combine all the ingredients.

Apply the mixture to your face, and let it sit for 15 to 20 minutes.

Rinse the mask off with warm water, a face wash, and a washcloth.

BEAUTY TIPS
to Refresh

- Sleep! Get your beauty rest!

- Do a face mask.

- Apply a hair mask.

- Do a total-body sugar or ground coffee scrub.

- Have a clean shave . . .
  no, but seriously, it feels so good.

- Have a mani-pedi.

- Exfoliate your lips
  (make a scrub with sugar and honey).

- Apply a deep moisturizer over your whole body.

- Place cucumber slices on your eyes.

- Apply peppermint oil to your wrists.

- Rub coconut oil . . . everywhere.

refresh

HOW TO FEEL REFRESHED AFTER A BREAKUP

The more you feel, the more you heal.

When you're going through a tough breakup, it can be tempting to head right for the ice cream and Netflix—but we want you to take care of yourself right now, because this is a time to prioritize *you*.

Over wine, healthy snacks, and some chocolate, we sat fireside with our girlfriends to hear their amazing advice, which we now share with you:

- Leave the "what ifs" behind. Start living in the "what is."

- It's easy to romanticize the good times, but remember why you're in this place to move forward with your life.

- If the breakup is new, we understand. If it was years ago and still feels bad, we get that too. Everyone heals in their own time.

- Avoid their Instagram and who's liking their pics or the photos they're tagged in. We know it's hard, but doing so will make the process easier.

- Don't worry about the time spent in that relationship— because it was something that you cared about. It made you into the strong person you are today, and it will only improve your standards for your life in the future.

- Find peace in knowing that if they're in a better place, you had a positive impact on their life. Even if it didn't work out, you made your ex a better person—you had a part in that.

- Remember to be kind to yourself. You've done everything you can, and there are no regrets, just lessons—always.

- Keep busy—really busy. This is a time to learn a new skill, take a fun class, schedule get-togethers, start training for a race you've been wanting to do, study for that certification you've been wanting to earn, or volunteer for a charity.

- It's good to go through all the emotions. Give yourself permission to feel so you can fully process what you're going through. It will make you stronger.

- Whatever it takes to make you feel good, do that. A lot of it.

- Inhale positivity; exhale what you don't want . . . every day.

- Find happiness in your independence. This is a chance to get to know yourself, rediscover the strong woman you are, and experience new things.

- Use a journal as a safe venting place to explore your feelings, what you learned from the relationship (good and bad!), and what you want to refocus on now.

- Explore new classes: boxing, yoga, Pilates, barre, dance—you just may find a new passion!

- Take a girls' trip or a little getaway. Yoga retreat? Yes, please!

- Fall in love with yourself again.

You *always* deserve the best! It can be easy to lose sight of this during a breakup, but you are worth it, you are phenomenal, you are freaking gorgeous, and you deserve incredible things along with a lifetime of happiness. You are strong, and you will get through this. And there is so much waiting for you just around the corner!

—xo, *Angela, Kerry, and Katie*

refresh

You've now had a chance to work out, try some yummy recipes and treatments, and receive the best girlfriend advice in the world. You're starting a healthy routine. Remember, you have a whole community from around the world to support you. Connect with new gal pals on Instagram through #TIUteam, or meet TIU girls in your area with #TIUyourcity or #TIUyourarea.

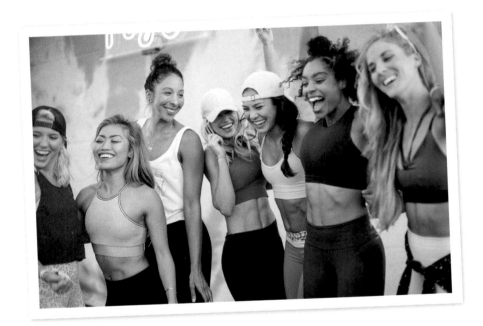

Real Women, Real Stories

"One time I donated the 'Forgive me' roses that showed up on my desk. They were so beautiful, but I just couldn't keep them. I dropped them off to people who would actually appreciate them on my way home—the children's hospital. It was so freeing."

—Angela

"I took a vase of roses from my doorstep and put them back on his . . . with a note that said 'Return to sender.' Oops."

—Katie

"I received the final rose . . . so I took a picture of the vase among the rest of the empty apology vases and posted it with the caption 'Spring Cleaning. Every vase has its story.'"

—Kerry

refresh

CONNECT WITH THE
TONE IT UP COMMUNITY
to Refresh

There is something so refreshing about spending time with our pals and nourishing our female friendships. We built this beautiful community so women could find good friends just like we did. Nothing makes us happier than seeing women connect and watching their friendships blossom—it's a dream come true for us. In the TIU community, women share stories with accountability partners, best friends, and even sisters. We are so proud to be a part of something that brings women together every day.

Stories from Community Members

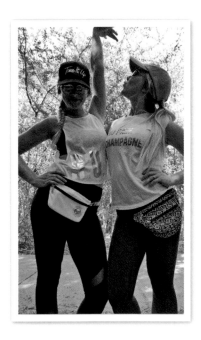

Kelly and Mandy

Kelly @kshupe and Mandy @tiu_mandy7

"Kelly and I first connected at a #TIUTexas meet-up! We were at a restaurant, and she was sitting across from me and had the most gorgeous mermaid waves. I'm pretty sure the first thing I ever said to her was asking how she got her hair to look like that! After that, we discovered that we lived only a few minutes from each other and that we went to the same gym. So naturally we started scheduling gym dates and started doing some classes together. We just clicked, and the rest is history!

"Kelly is constantly encouraging me. One time that comes to mind is actually right before the TIU Tour. I had ordered some leggings to wear to the tour, and I was so excited! But when I received them and tried them on, I was not happy about the way they fit. Suddenly, just from one pair of leggings, I was picking my body apart. Kelly told me that I was beautiful and how proud she was of me for how hard I've worked and how far I've come. Just hearing her say that made me feel so much better. It reminded me that our perceptions of ourselves are sometimes not what others see. I ditched those pants and found a new outfit and felt so confident at the tour!"

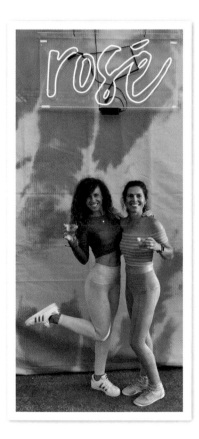

Sarah and Betsy

Sarah @tiusarie and Betsy @tiubetsy

"Sarah and I first connected at the 2016 TIU Retreat in Dana Point. After such a magical time, I went home dreaming of creating an amazing group of TIU Arizona babes! I reached out to Sarah as soon as I got back home!

"Sarah and I usually plan our meetups together in Scottsdale. We have planned some fun hikes, coffee dates, shopping dates at Kendra Scott, and delicious meals at our favorite place to eat, True Foods! We also got to do life together when I road-tripped it down to

refresh

her house for a couple of days. We did a fun girls' night and dressed up and spent the night talking about all the fun things we have in common. It's so amazing and magical to find your person who you know you can just count on and get to experience all the things that make you happy—together!"

Jamey and Jessy

Jamey @tiu_jamey and Jessy @jessyjean_tiu

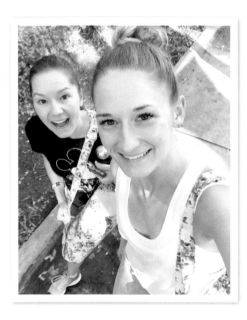

"We first found each other on Instagram in the #TIUcommunity and then connected through the #TIUDFW group chat. After a few weeks, we soon realized that we lived *right* down the street from each other. So on a random Sunday, we decided to meet up at a new local juice bar in our area to connect in person with each other! We hit it off right away, talking for hours over green juices about how we started with Tone It Up, our fitness goals, and our life stories! From that point forward, we knew we would become #TIUbesties!

"In reflecting on our journey together thus far, we are stronger, more motivated, and happier because we have found each other. It is through Tone It Up that we had the opportunity to connect, meet, and fall in love with taking care of our bodies through fitness together. We prep together, plan workouts together, talk on the regular to keep each other on track, and have found our fitness soul sisters in each other! We are so thankful to have come this far and know we wouldn't be where we are without our other half right there next to us believing in us through it all.

"We have grown emotionally into positive, happy people. We have grown physically in strength and endurance, because having that other person beside you, pushing just as hard through a workout, helps you take that extra inch, that extra rep, and that extra exhale—and in the long run makes you that much stronger. We are like-minded, fitness-oriented, and health-driven individuals that are able to be our true, raw, and authentic selves around each other because we are constantly building each other up and trust one another with our whole hearts. We have seen each other's sweatiest of sweats, celebrated each other's highest of highs, and picked each other up at our lows. We can be silly, serious, and sweaty all at the same time!"

Camryn and Calyn

Camryn @tropi_cam
and Calyn @cayy_tiu

Camryn and Calyn are twin sisters and TIU accountability partners!

"Camryn first discovered Tone It Up on YouTube. She got started by following the workouts for a few months but was still struggling with nutrition. Her #TIUboyfriend gave

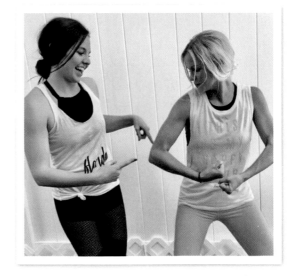

refresh

her the Nutrition Plan as a Christmas gift and everything changed after that! Watching her reach her goals and be a total boss babe made me want to join Tone It Up too! We immediately felt a sense of connection to Tone It Up after first discovering them because just like K&K we are Cay&Cam. We love the bond that they share, as it feels similar to ours. We know that, like them, we can do so much more when we love and support each other!" —*Cay*

"We set goals and get to reach them together! It's amazing to share something so special that we are both passionate about. Tone It Up has enhanced our bond as sisters and given us a common appreciation for our health and wellness!" —*Cam*

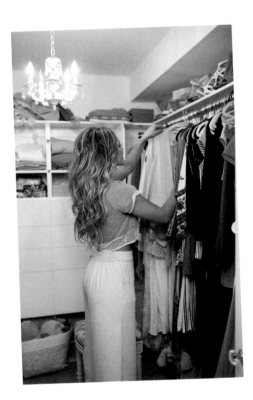

ACTION GUIDE
to Refresh

KATRINA   Imagine your space completely clean—your closet, kitchen, bedroom, bathroom, that junk drawer. You can do a spring cleaning no matter what the season. It's one of the best ways to bring new energy into your home while letting go of things you don't need. Once it's gone, you'll have more space for all the goals you'll achieve!

Just a few weeks ago, our girlfriends Angela and Kerry were moving into their new place, and they needed some help—actually, everyone always needs help when they move. So my advice: always show up with a lending hand for your friends! Moving is a perfect opportunity to cleanse your closet. So after we moved everything in, I grabbed a bottle of wine, played some old school jams, and made some healthy snacks so we could get after it. We started with Angela's clothes, which she hadn't gone through in years—I may have found multiple cutoffs from our spring break trip! The trick to letting things go seamlessly is to hold up the piece of clothing for her and ask, "Have you worn this in the last year? If you went shopping today, would you buy it? And most important, do you feel confident in it, and will you actually wear it?" If the answer is yes, hang it up! If not, it's time to say goodbye. And if something is really special and sentimental—like a scarf your grandmother knit for you—of course you need to keep it. I still have the sweatshirt I was wearing when Brian proposed to me. It was already falling apart when I wore it, but I can't seem to let it go. I like to say that I'm sentimental—not a hoarder! After all the music, wine, and snacks, Angela and Kerry ended up donating more than half of their closets and didn't miss a thing—not even their high school cheer shorts. They

refresh

said they wouldn't have been able to do it if they had held up every piece themselves. Plus, a lot of the clothing was business casual from previous jobs, so we filled six large bags and brought them to a women's shelter for those who may really need it.

Tips to Refresh Your Home

CLOSET

Color coordinate! We swear by it. It's a total life changer, because when you know you want to wear that coral sweater, you know exactly where to find it. We also go through our workout clothes every few months. If you don't see yourself grabbing those capris, donate them. Remember, when you feel confident during your workout, you always run the extra mile! Organize your sports bras, let go of old socks, and make it easier than ever to grab your workout clothes on busy mornings. I actually have my sports bras and socks in little fabric baskets at the bottom of my closet, instead of in a drawer, so I can just grab them. I roll my yoga pants and put them in a basket too, so I can see which ones I'm grabbing.

PANTRY AND FRIDGE

In the kitchen, sort through and organize the shelves, pantry, fridge, and freezer separately. The first things to go are anything that's old or expired. Even spices go stale, so toss them when in doubt. For each food item, ask yourself, "Is this food good for me, and does it help me reach my fitness goals?" If the answer is no, it's time to get rid of it or to donate the nonperishables. (If it's something your husband or kids can't live without, move it to a different cabinet that you don't open every day.) If you find cooking utensils and appliances that will help you cook easy and healthy meals, like a blender or food processor, buried in the back of your cabinets, move them to easily accessible spots. You can also organize your Tupperware (find all those matching lids!), and set mason jars aside to make meal prep a breeze.

BEAUTY PRODUCTS

Go through those drawers, and let go of anything you don't use. We all accumulate makeup and hair products, but those go bad too. After you've gone through everything, wash your makeup brushes. It feels *ahh*-mazing!

Here's how: Fill a small cup with lukewarm water and a drop of gentle soap or baby shampoo. Gently swirl the brush tips in the cup, then rinse them under running water. Squeeze out any excess moisture and reshape the bristles, then lay your brushes flat to air-dry. Quick and easy! I actually bring them into the shower with me in a cup while I shampoo too—no shame in the game, ha-ha!

YOUR RIDE

Workin' at the car wash, yeah! Time to go through your car and make space for that inspiring commute. If you have to drive a lot, make your car a mini sanctuary for yourself. Get a supportive back pillow; pack a mini makeup bag with lip balm, sunscreen, and elastics for your center console; download podcasts for your ride; make playlists for inspiration while you drive; and clean out the clutter that could be stressing you out.

One of the very best things about cleaning up is that you can always find someone or someplace that can use your items, so nothing will go to waste. We donate to our local Salvation Army, Goodwill, or any other nearby drop-off center or women's shelter. There are also many

refresh

great organizations, like One World Running and Soles4Soles, which collect and repurpose old running shoes. And local food banks are always in need of nonperishable food donations.

Last, but not least . . .

REFRESH YOUR MIND

It's so much easier to get caught up in the things that aren't working, plans falling through, disappointments, and daily stress. Every day we have so many worries that it's actually hard to focus on the positive—it takes work to shift our minds, real work. When we see only the negative, we develop an emotional disconnection, we lose our creativity,

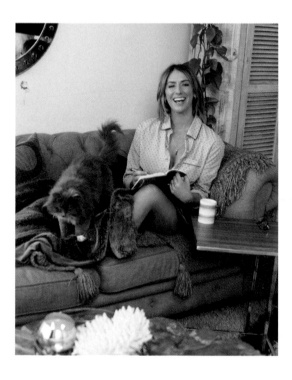

and we feel defeated. Negative thoughts affect the entire body too—cortisol levels rise, causing stomach fat; the neck tenses up; blood pressure rises; and headaches, irritability, or insomnia can develop. We're going to put all that behind us!

We want you to pick up a pen and write down five things that you're going to let go from your mind. This could be anything that doesn't serve you: toxic thoughts and conversations, negative self-talk, an unhealthy relationship, fears that hold you back from achieving

SIMPLE WAYS TO
FEEL REFRESHED

We asked our girlfriends how they feel refreshed . . .

- Walk outside in the fresh air.

- Open the curtains and windows.

- Take a nap in the sun.

- Take a bubble bath.

- Do a yoga class.

- Have a facial.

- Put freshly cut flowers in your home.

- Get some new undies and socks—totally underrated.

- Put clean sheets on the bed . . . seriously, the best. (Putting on the duvet cover counts as a workout too. Bonus points for folding a fitted sheet!)

- Take three cleansing breaths—with grapefruit essential oil.

- Rearrange a room.

- Add some new accent pillows.

your dreams. Any time you find these thoughts popping into your mind, think back to this list and your intention to let it go. The more you release negativity and worry, the more space you have to embrace new challenges, positivity, and love.

From here on out, instead of focusing on what is happening to you, focus on what is happening *for you!* Make one more list of five things that are happening *for you.* It could be your health, a great friendship, access to healthy foods, an education, or a promotion at work. Recognize what is great, and jot it down.

refresh

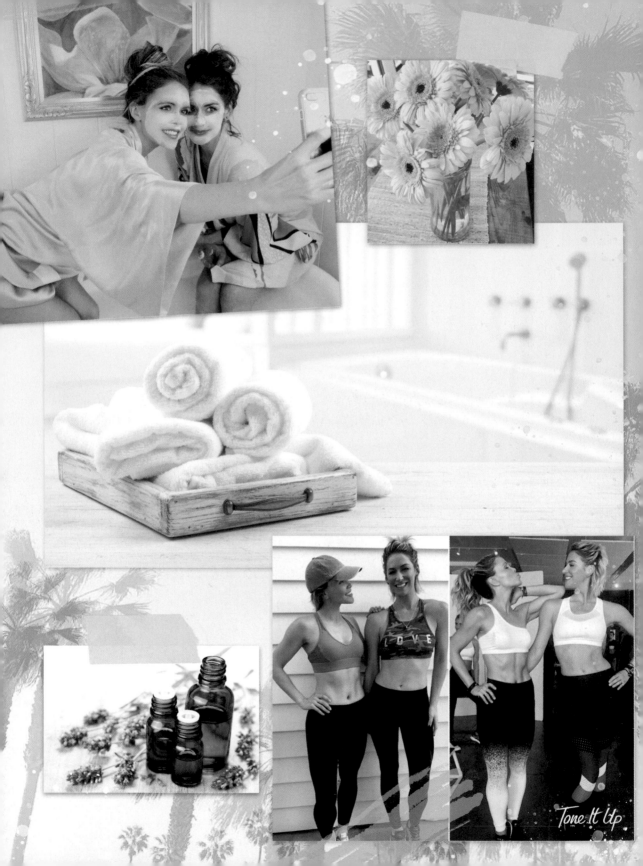

Tone It Up

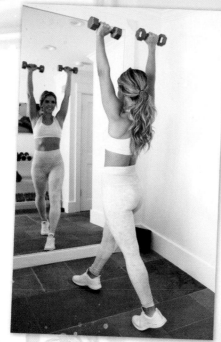

Vision Board to Refresh

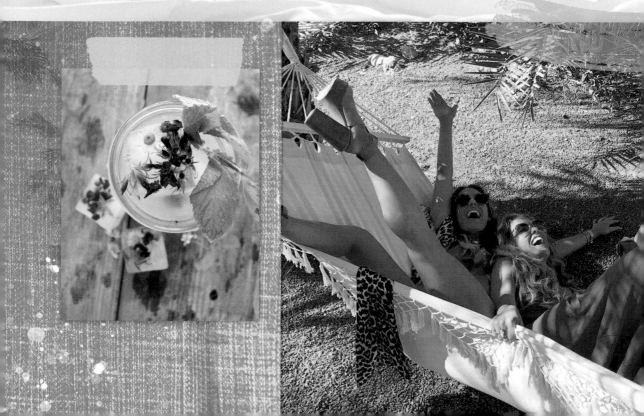

REFLECT
to Refresh

I feel most refreshed when I

_____

An exercise I can do to feel refreshed is

_____

A time in my past when I really needed to feel refreshed was

_____

If I could do one thing to feel more refreshed right now it would be

_____

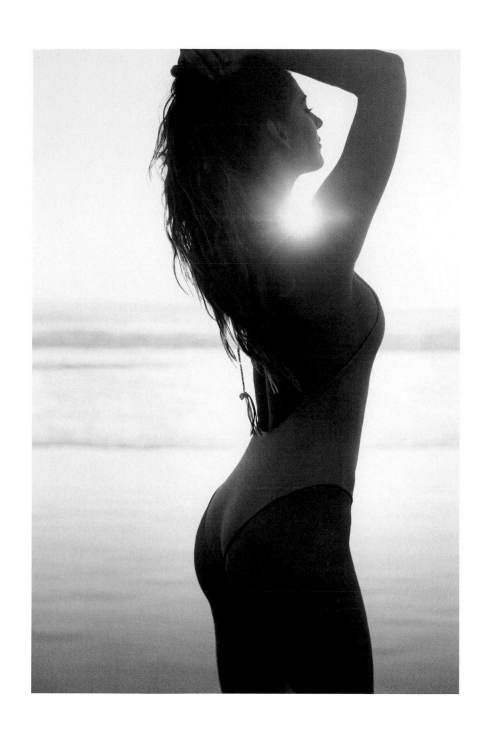

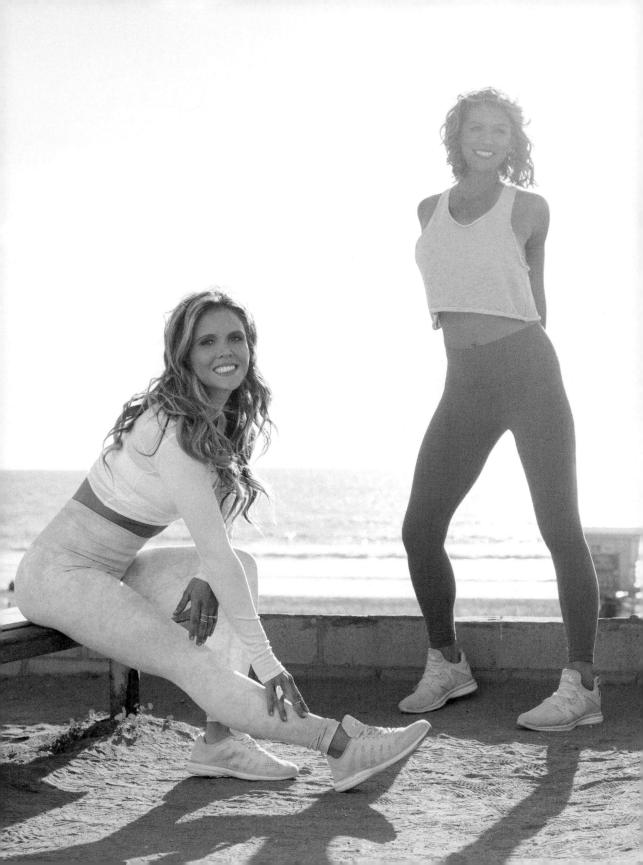

2

Motivate

Be fearless in the pursuit of what sets your soul on fire.

—UNKNOWN

GIRL TALK
to Motivate

KATRINA   I'm going to share something that may surprise you. If you've been following Tone It Up and our journey, you may think that we're always motivated, but we find ourselves in lulls too, when life gets in the way, and time will pass when we haven't done anything for our personal growth, our spiritual growth, or our physical well-being in what feels like forever.

I have an all-or-nothing type of personality, which can be good and bad. In a good way, I'm all in and you can always count on me to make something great. In a bad way, I start neglecting other parts of my life that may need some love and care (shout-out to my amazing husband, who has stood by me through a lot of this!). I'm aware of my faults, and recognition is a strength. If I slip up, I know I don't have to wait until Monday to start again, and if I mess up something with work, the project isn't completely lost. I've noticed that when I lose myself, it's usually because I'm focused on making something perfect. I completely devote myself to a project or even sometimes to helping someone on their journey, then I lose myself and my own motivation. If a friend is in need, I'll drop everything (and I'd do so again right now!), which isn't all bad, but it's something I need to keep in mind when it comes to my health. Working on myself inside can show up externally. Finding balance has taken me a long time—and I'm still working on it each day.

We all go through it—dips in motivation and slip-ups—but if I've learned anything on my journey, *the comeback is always greater than the setback.* That's for sure!

47

Karena and I sat down with our girlfriends last night and asked them how they find motivation, and it was the same across the board: we find it in each other! Whenever we're getting ready for an event or a trip, or we want to get back on track, we confide in each other. We book workouts together for the week, meal prep together, and share our goals to hold one another accountable. That's why the community is so powerful!

Karena is a major source of motivation for me. Since we met, she's been my number one supporter and biggest cheerleader. I'll always go to her when I feel like I need a pep talk—or if I need to confess something. She and I will actually have a full-on confessional. We're like "*Okay, that's enough. This weekend I had too many treats, and today I'm a new woman!*" or "*Confession: It's been seven days and four and a half hours since I touched a weight . . . but I need you to check up on me later and make sure I do today's daily moves.*" Together, we plan our schedule and sign up for workouts in Studio Tone It Up and at our favorite yoga spots. We have a shared calendar, which helps a lot. And if we're not going to a class together, we still check in with each other. If you create a shared workout calendar with a girlfriend, it's major motivation!

Where can you find motivation? Think about what ignites you. What makes your heart beat faster even thinking about it? What do you want to make a priority in your life? Is it a passion of yours? Is it that girl you imagine yourself becoming with every choice you make? We want you to be great. We want you to be your most powerful, authentic, badass superbabe self. And the way to get there is to visualize her every day!

For us, the Tone It Up community is what sets our souls on fire. All we need to do is look at the brilliant and beautiful women of this team— and it's you who make our hearts beat faster. You're our motivation to work hard each and every day, so we have you to thank.

What Motivates Me

What personally motivates me is achieving a positive result from hard work. In my early teens and early twenties, I struggled deeply and finally realized I wasn't living my best life. I listened to that small voice within me that told me that this was not how my life was meant to be. I listened even harder and found the motivation and perseverance to overcome and *become* who I really am. It was a time of awakening. This can be true in all aspects of life: work, love, friendships, spirituality, and your inner self.

I believe we all have the power to find our purpose and passion. We just have to let go, listen, and lead our lives.

Karena

What Motivates Me

I've always been a super-passionate person, so I use that as a tool to find motivation. I'm constantly thinking about what I want to achieve next and how I can get there. I journal everything and use the power of visualization to get me there. It began when I was in the sixth grade and started journaling, writing down my goals and workouts, running and lifting weights. I manifested the life I wanted, worked hard, and saw my life take shape and transform. Looking back, I realize I was in the driver's seat of my life, and I wasn't stuck in something that didn't feel like me. Knowing that has empowered me and made me feel like I can do anything I set my heart to. I'm also motivated by my girlfriends, my family, my husband Brian, and this community. I love seeing the people I care about take their passion and use it to propel themselves forward.

Katrina

motivate

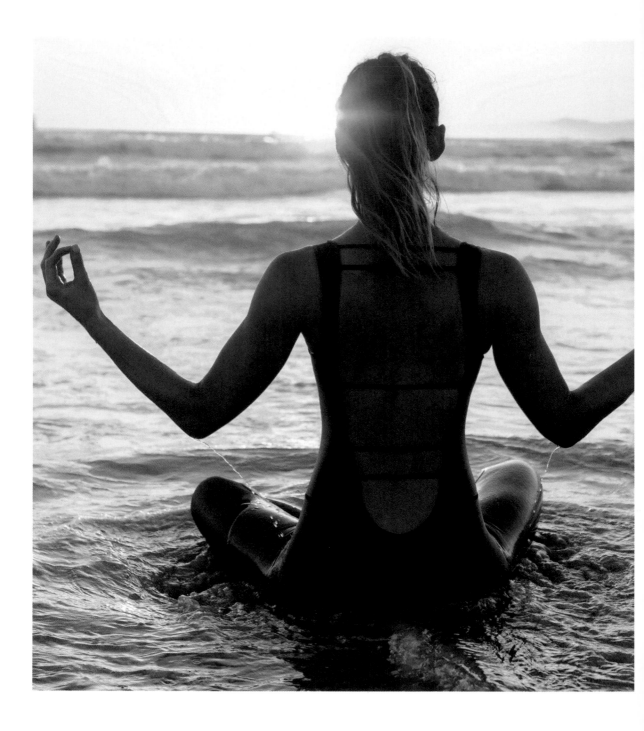

SPIRITUAL GUIDE
to Motivate

KARENA After years of meditating and devoting myself to personal growth, I took my first training in transcendental meditation (TM). I offer guided meditations on ToneItUp.com and on our app—from perseverance to grounding, strength, peace, and self-love. When most people think of meditation, they picture lying on a mat with their eyes closed, in Savasana. But that's just one form of meditation. Meditation can be anything that calms, relaxes, and centers you, whether done while moving or while remaining still. It can be running, cooking, boxing, swimming, hiking, playing a musical instrument, tennis, drawing, making floral arrangements—anything you do while also connecting to your breath and your thoughts. Whatever form it takes, let it be just you and your mind—with no judgment or expectations, simply your effortless presence and pure being. When you are present and connected in your body, and all that's left is your breath and mindful thoughts, *that* is meditation.

Letting go of distractions and truly focusing on your body can be a challenge—especially if your mind is running a mile a minute. It's a challenge for us too! We've learned that when we quiet our minds for those few minutes, we're so much more productive and focused for the rest of the day. Research shows that daily meditation can lead to increased activity in the prefrontal cortex of the brain, which helps regulate stress. It can also help lower production of the stress hormone cortisol and boost self-confidence and optimism.

The following are some steps of the simplest form of meditation. Start with meditating just a few minutes and work your way up to

51

more. It will begin to feel natural and become an amazing part of your routine that you look forward to every morning. Pretty soon, you'll discover your favorite form of mindful meditation—something you love that puts your mind at ease. The next time you do something you love, pay attention to where your thoughts lead you. You'll discover deeper states of consciousness and live more fully and with intent— one of the best feelings ever!

- Find a quiet, comfortable place to sit. No distractions.

- Before you start, decide how long you want to meditate. It can be from five to ten minutes or longer if you have the time. Set a timer so you don't need to keep glancing at a clock or wonder if time has passed too quickly.

- We recommend listening to meditation music or soothing sounds that you can download onto your phone.

- Close your eyes and take three deep cleansing breaths. With each breath, fill your lungs for a count of five, holding at the peak of each inhale before exhaling slowly, either through your nose or mouth. Allow your breathing to return to normal, and start observing each breath. This is all you have to do. Focus your attention on your heart, and truly feel what it's like to simply be with yourself.

- Be present and aware of whatever sensations come up, and let them wash over you. If there are noises around you or feelings of restlessness coming up, just let them be. It's best not to resist anything. Your mind may be racing nonstop, and that's okay. Keep breathing, and when you remember, bring your awareness back to your heart.

- While you're meditating, try thinking of three words of intention that you feel you need *now*. It could be love, gratitude, presence, peace, nonjudgment. Silently think of these words throughout your meditation, and recall them during the rest of your day. Do this and then watch the magic unfold.

- If your mind wanders, as it inevitably will, don't judge yourself. This is part of the meditation. Gently and lovingly bring your attention back to your breath and to your heart. (The more you meditate, the easier it will be to focus.) Continue this rhythm until the time is up.

- At the end of your allotted time, don't get up right away. Turn off the timer (if you're using one) and keep your eyes closed. Take three deep breaths, and open your eyes when it feels right. It's sometimes nice to sit for a few minutes afterward to collect your thoughts and reinforce your intentions.

- Take that feeling of calmness and awareness with you throughout the rest of your day.

How to Set Up a Meditation Space

You don't need a dedicated place to meditate if you're short on space, but it should be a spot in your home where you can sit comfortably. You may like to lie down on a yoga mat, while others like to sit in a comfy chair or on a sofa. You might want to dim the lights or put on a sleep mask. The most important thing is that this space is calm, quiet, and soothing for you.

For more ideas, see "Create an Inspiration Area in Your Home" on page 98, in the "Inspire" chapter.

Mindful Evenings to Motivate You

Most of us lose steam by the end of the day. To keep yourself motivated and on top of your goals, get organized before you settle in.

Also, when you're getting ready for bed, do a mindful run-through of everything you accomplished that day, big or small. Every little thing is significant.

Take a quick look at your motivation list too. What did you do well today? *Any* steps you took toward your goals are meaningful and important. State your goals again, to help you creatively visualize them. Yes, you are going to reach your goals!

DAILY DEVOTIONS

KARENA I like to start each day reading a devotion from *A Year of Miracles* by Marianne Williamson. It helps me feel centered and sets my intention for the day ahead. These are a couple of reflections I find myself returning to:

Our very cells respond to the thoughts we think. With every word, silent or spoken, we participate in the body's functioning. We participate in the functioning of the universe itself. If our consciousness grows lighter, then so does everything within and around us. This means, of course, that with every thought, we can start to re-create our lives. In saying yes to new beginnings, we begin to bring them forth.

I am open to change and I will not resist it. I will not resist what occurs today. I open my heart to new places, new people, and new chapters of my life.

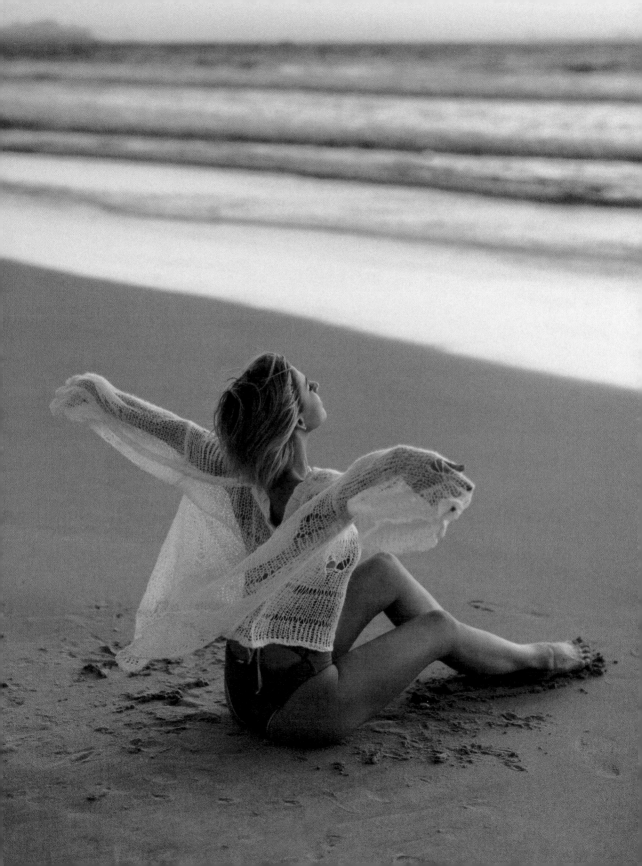

MAKE A MOTIVATION LIST
AND
VISUALIZE YOUR SUCCESS

KATRINA We love our lists! A motivation list is a great tool to help you pinpoint what motivates you and what will keep you motivated. So we have a challenge for you right now: grab your favorite journal and pen and create your own motivation list as you read this. This will be a powerful exercise. Let's all do it together!

- The first step is to define what you want. Close your eyes and visualize how you want to feel. Are you healthy and energized? Toned and strong? Fulfilled in your career and relationships? Pursuing a new passion? Exuding positivity? More confident than ever? Whatever it is, open your eyes and write it down. When you physically write down your motivations, you're telling yourself: *"I promise you this."* This makes your mind go to work on helping you stick to the plan.

- When you're writing out your list, be positive. Focus on what you want to accomplish, not what you want to get rid of. For example, instead of setting a goal of losing 10 pounds, be motivated to be healthy by exercising daily. Instead of not feeling tired anymore, make it your goal to have tons of energy through eating healthy foods and getting plenty of sleep and hydration.

- Now that you have your list of goals, it's time to picture yourself where you want to be. All you need to do is imagine yourself achieving your goals: visualize yourself getting stronger, running longer distances, and pursuing your passions. Athletes use visualization all the time, and

Karena and I have used it to reach goals in our own lives. Use visualization while meditating, during workouts, right when you wake up, or when you're about to fall asleep at night. It really works!

We have no doubt that you can alter your circumstances and increase your happiness with your motivation list and positive visualization. This is about believing and seeing yourself get where you want to be. It's about envisioning what your motivation is and focusing on your thoughts and dreams to make them into reality. This is true for your health, your career, your relationships, your friendships—all aspects of your life!

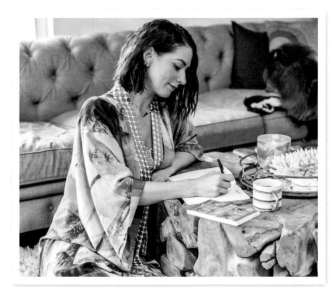

motivate

WORKOUT GUIDE
to Motivate

You know what's motivating? Feeling strong, empowered, and fiercer than ever! That's how we feel after an upper body workout. There's something so powerful about gaining strength in your shoulders, back, and arms. Your posture is improved, you stand taller, and you lead your life with your heart.

Motivating Up Top

For this routine, use 5- to 10-pound weights. You can also do our fave, drop sets (as described on page 6), where you start with heavier weights and reduce the weights as you go.

Do *three circuits* of the following:

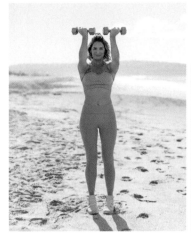
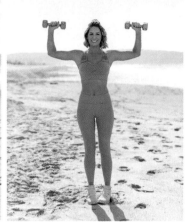
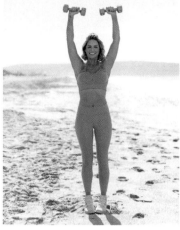

Arnold Press

15 REPS

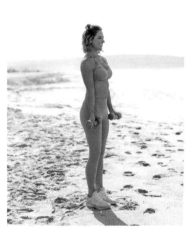
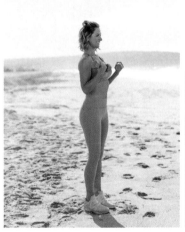
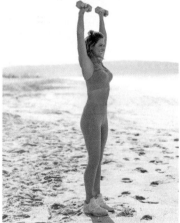

Biceps Curl to Press

15 REPS

motivate

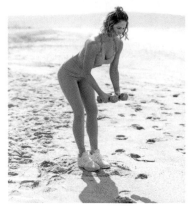
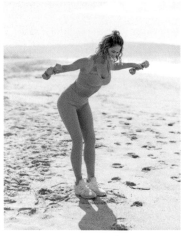

3

Reverse Fly

15 REPS

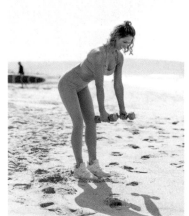
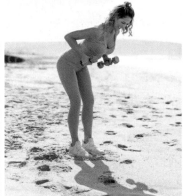
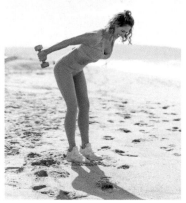

4

Row with Triceps Kickback

15 REPS

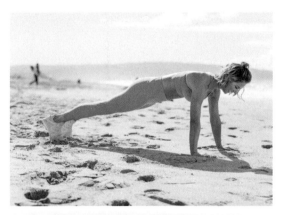

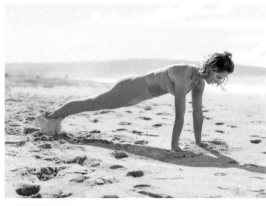

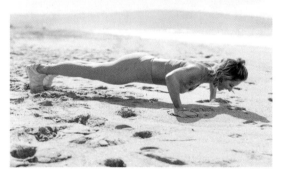

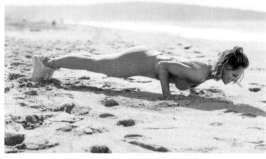

5 *Wide Arm Push-Up*

IO REPS

6 *Triceps Push-Up*

IO REPS

motivate

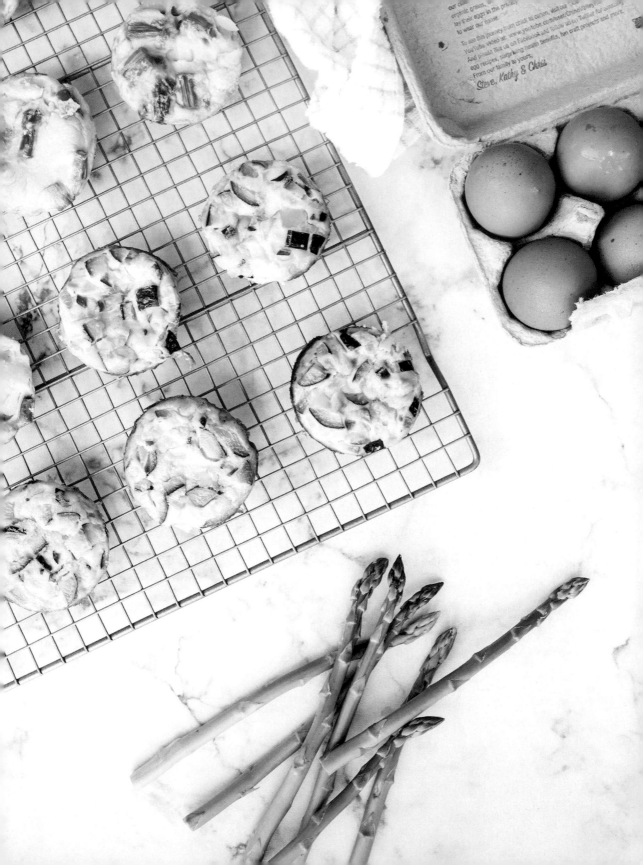

RECIPE GUIDE
to Motivate

There's no denying, a healthy meal can make you feel like Superwoman! It's so motivating to nourish your body the way it deserves. Choose some of the following favorite recipes to feel fabulous!

MORNING EGG BITES

Makes 12 (3 per serving)

We love these egg muffins! They're perfect to prep on a Sunday for use during the week.

Coconut oil spray
6 eggs
3 egg whites (or ½ cup)
Pinch of salt

1 cup chopped veggies of your choice (We love asparagus, spinach, peppers, onions, jalapeños, and mushrooms!)

Preheat the oven to 350°F.

Prep a mini muffin tin by coating it with the coconut oil spray.

In a mixing bowl, whisk together the eggs, egg whites, and salt, then stir in the vegetables.

Pour the egg mixture into the mini muffin tin, making sure to scoop some vegetables into each egg bite.

Bake the egg bites for 20 to 25 minutes.

After the egg bites have cooled, store them in a glass container in the fridge. They will keep for up to four days.

STRAWBERRY AVO-TOAST

Serves 1

2 slices whole wheat,
Ezekiel, or
gluten-free bread

½ avocado, peeled,
pitted, and mashed

4 strawberries,
stemmed and sliced

Honey

Sea salt

Toast the bread, then spread the slices with the mashed avocado.

Top the avocado with the sliced strawberries.

Drizzle the toast with honey, and add a dash of sea salt to each.

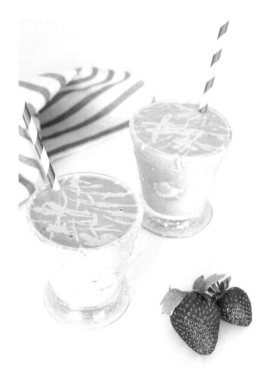

PB&J SMOOTHIE

Serves 1

10 ounces unsweetened almond milk

1 scoop vanilla Tone It Up Protein

½ cup frozen strawberries

½ frozen banana

1 tablespoon peanut butter

In a high-speed blender, blend all the ingredients until the mixture is smooth, and enjoy!

BLUEBERRY CHIA MUFFINS

Makes 6

Coconut oil spray

3/4 cup oat flour or
almond meal

3/4 cup vanilla
Tone It Up Protein

1 tablespoon chia seeds

1 teaspoon baking powder

1/2 teaspoon
ground cinnamon

1/4 teaspoon salt

1 egg

1/2 cup unsweetened
almond milk or coconut milk

2 tablespoons coconut oil,
melted

2 tablespoons maple syrup

1 teaspoon vanilla extract

1/2 cup frozen blueberries

Preheat the oven to 350°F.

Prep a muffin tin by coating it with the coconut oil spray.

In a mixing bowl, combine the flour or meal, Tone It Up Protein, chia seeds, baking powder, cinnamon, and salt.

In a separate bowl, lightly whisk the egg, then stir in the almond or coconut milk, melted coconut oil, maple syrup, and vanilla extract.

Stir the wet ingredients into the dry ingredients and mix well. Gently fold in the blueberries.

Pour the batter into the prepared tin, then bake the muffins for 20 to 25 minutes, or until they are lightly browned but not dry.

motivate

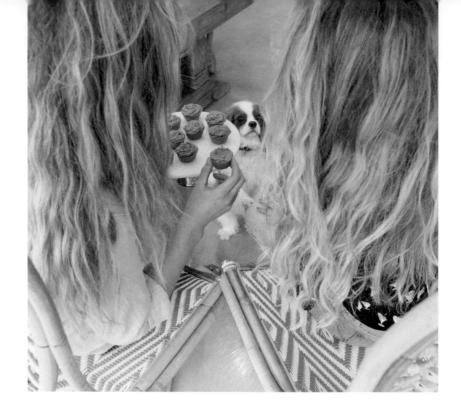

BLONDIE MUFFINS

Makes 12 mini muffins (3 per serving)

Coconut oil spray

1 15-ounce can chickpeas, drained and rinsed

1/2 cup unsweetened almond butter

1/4 teaspoon baking powder

1/4 teaspoon baking soda

1/2 teaspoon salt

1/4 cup maple syrup

2 teaspoons vanilla

Preheat the oven to 350°F.

Prepare a mini muffin tin by coating it with the coconut oil spray.

Puree all the ingredients in a food processor or a blender, then pour the batter into the prepared tin.

Bake the muffins for 18 to 20 minutes, or until a toothpick comes out clean.

K&K KALE SALAD
with LEMON ZEST DRESSING

Serves 3

To make this salad a main dish, you can top it with any lean protein of your choosing. Note that for easy eating and enjoying, you can chop any salad greens with kitchen shears!

4 cups stemmed and chopped kale

2 bell peppers, chopped

1/2 red onion, chopped

1/4 cup pine nuts

1 small bunch fresh cilantro, large stems removed, chopped

FOR THE DRESSING

Juice of 2 lemons

Zest of 1 lemon

2 tablespoons grapeseed oil

2 tablespoons agave syrup

Pinch of Himalayan pink salt

Toss the kale, bell peppers, onion, pine nuts, and cilantro together in a bowl.

In a separate bowl, whisk together all the dressing ingredients, then pour the dressing over the salad and serve.

motivate

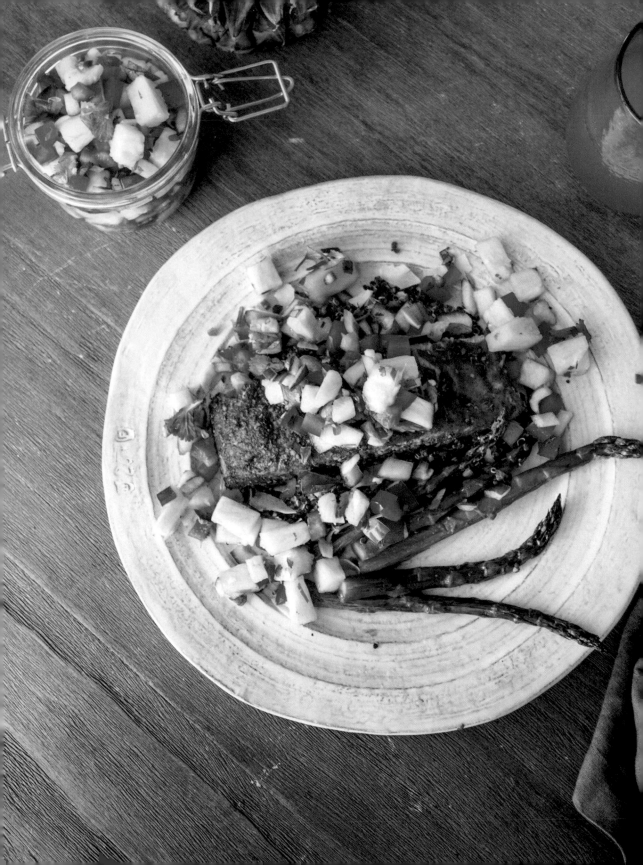

BLACKENED SALMON
with PINEAPPLE SALSA

Serves 1

You will have enough leftover Pineapple Salsa for an additional serving, which you'll need for Day 4's menu (page 157). This spicy-sweet salsa can keep in the fridge for up to four days.

1 tablespoon ground paprika

1 teaspoon garlic granules

1 teaspoon dried thyme

Pinch of ground cayenne

1/4 teaspoon ground black pepper

6 ounces salmon

Coconut oil spray

FOR THE SALSA

1/4 cup chopped fresh pineapple

1/4 cup chopped bell pepper

1 jalapeño, seeded and diced

1/2 cup diced red onion

Juice of 1 lime

Pinch of salt

Preheat the oven to 375°F.

In a bowl, combine the blackening seasoning: the paprika, garlic granules, thyme, cayenne, and black pepper. Rub the seasoning onto all sides of the salmon.

Coat a baking sheet with the coconut oil spray, then place the seasoned salmon on the sheet and bake it for 25 to 30 minutes, or until the salmon is firm but not dry.

While the salmon is baking, prepare the salsa. Combine all the salsa ingredients in a bowl, and let the flavors meld at room temperature until the salmon is ready. Top the cooked salmon with half the salsa, and reserve the other half in the fridge.

motivate

TIU TRAY BAKE

Serves 1

Double or triple the recipe for more servings during the week.

½ cup chopped yellow onion

2 to 3 garlic cloves, chopped

2 teaspoons olive oil

1 tablespoon chili powder (optional)

1 tablespoon curry powder (optional)

1 teaspoon lemon pepper (optional)

¼ teaspoon ground cayenne (optional)

Pinch of salt

VEGGIES (CHOOSE UP TO THREE FROM THE LIST)

1 cup halved brussels sprouts

1 cup chopped carrots

1 cup chopped green beans

½ cup cubed sweet potato or winter squash (acorn, butternut, delicata, pumpkin)

1 cup chopped fennel bulb

1 cup chopped cauliflower

1 cup chopped broccoli

1 cup chopped asparagus

PROTEIN (CHOOSE ONE FROM THE LIST)

6 ounces chicken breast

6 ounces salmon

6 ounces whitefish

6 ounces shrimp

½ cup canned beans, drained and rinsed (chickpea, pinto, black, kidney, navy)

Preheat the oven to 375°F.

On a baking sheet, toss all the ingredients together, making sure everything gets coated in the spices and oil.

Bake for 20 to 40 minutes, depending on your protein choice, but about halfway through the cooking, turn the vegetables to make sure everything is cooking evenly.

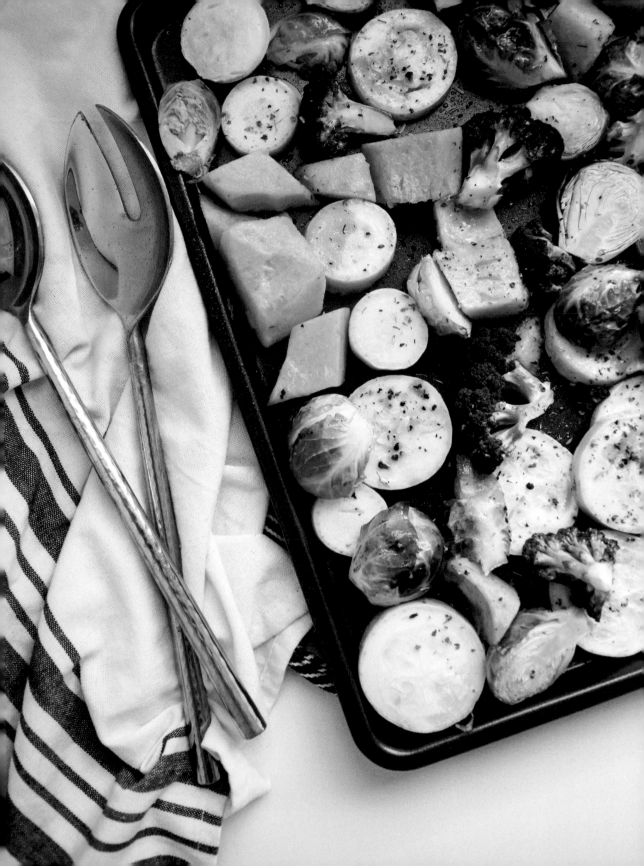

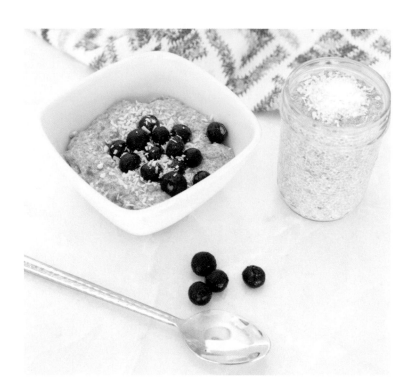

TOASTED COCONUT
CHIA PUDDING

Serves 3

¼ cup chia seeds

1 cup toasted-coconut
almond milk

Pinch of salt

Berries of your choice
(optional)

Unsweetened toasted
coconut flakes (optional)

Combine all the ingredients in a bowl, then divide the mixture into
serving bowls or jars, and allow them to sit in the fridge for 1 to 2 hours
to set.

If desired, serve the puddings topped with your favorite berries and/
or coconut flakes.

GIRLFRIEND GUIDE
to Motivate

The Power of Accountability

Having an accountability partner will be the most motivating and powerful decision you can make on your journey. With a girlfriend by your side, you're even stronger, you're unstoppable, and you can achieve absolutely anything together. Research shows that having a network of friends and accountability partners helps you achieve your goals:

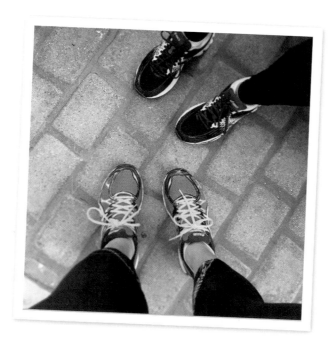

motivate

- A study from the *British Journal of Health Psychology*[1] shows that people who exercise with friends work out more regularly, and their friends motivate them in their sweat sessions, especially when those friends offer emotional support and encouragement. Gimme workout buddies!

- In an ongoing series of studies from Northwestern University,[2] researchers found that people who participate in social communities aimed at healthier living are more successful in reaching their goals.

- In a 2015 University of Pennsylvania study,[3] people who actively participated in a social media network went to more exercise classes and drastically improved their fitness levels over a thirteen-week period. Hello, #TIUteam on the 'gram!

Any time you have a goal, share it with someone who supports you. Or even better, ask them to do it with you. Check out the clubs or sports leagues in your area and join them. Kickball or volleyball anyone? And of course, if you haven't already, join the Tone It Up community. It's full of kind, welcoming women who are eager to support you and get to know you.

1 Pamela Rackow, Urte Scholz, and Rainer Hornung, "Received Social Support and Exercising: An Intervention Study to Test the Enabling Hypothesis," *British Journal of Health Psychology* 20, no. 5 (November 2015): 763–76, https://doi.org/10.1111/bjhp.12139.

2 J. Poncela-Casasnovas, B. Spring, D. McClary, A. C. Moller, R. Mukogo, C. A. Pellegrini, M. J. Coons, M. Davidson, S. Mukherjee, and L. A. Nunes Amaral, "Social Embeddedness in an Online Weight Management Programme Is Linked to Greater Weight Loss," *Journal of the Royal Society Interface* 12, no. 104 (March 6, 2015), doi: 10.1098/rsif.2014.0686.

3 Jingwen Zhang, Devon Brackbill, Sijia Yang, and Damon Centola, "Efficacy and Causal Mechanism of an Online Social Media Intervention to Increase Physical Activity: Results of a Randomized Controlled Trial," *Preventive Medicine Reports* 2 (2015): 651–57, doi: 10.1016/j.pmedr.2015.08.005; Jingwen Zhang, Devon Brackbill, Sijia Yang, and Damon Centola, "Identifying the Effects of Social Media on Health Behavior: Data from a Large-Scale Online Experiment," *Data in Brief* 5 (2015): 453–57, http://ndg.asc.upenn.edu/wp-content/uploads/2016/04/Zhang-2015-DIB.pdf.

BEAUTY TIPS
to Motivate

Whether we're headed to an intense workout or going to a meeting and want to feel super motivated, we're always rockin' at least three of the following:

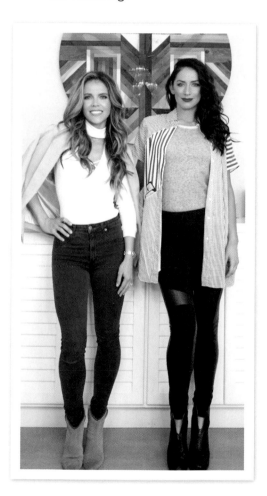

- Brow game—strong

- Slicked back hair

- Cute workout outfit
  (You may even lift more!)

- A good highlighter
  on the cheekbones

- Power-red lips

- Power heels

- Structured shoulders
  in a top for
  a meeting or event

motivate

CONNECT WITH THE TONE IT UP COMMUNITY
to Motivate

Some days you may feel a surge of motivation and believe there's nothing you can't do. And then you have those days, like we all do, when even a simple workout feels like moving a mountain—and it's totally okay. For the days when you need extra motivation, it's more important than ever to turn to your friends, your community, and your trainers for a pick-me-up. We asked some of the most motivating women we know—your amazing trainers from our Studio Tone It Up app—what they personally do when they need a little boost. These women are inspiring mega babes, and they continually motivate us!

Stories from Community Members

Stefanie

Stefanie, HIIT and strength trainer for Studio Tone It Up, @studiotoneitupstefanie

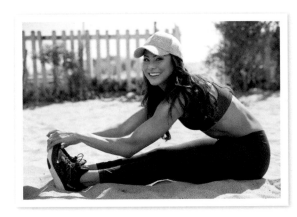

"I call a friend for a workout date! My excuses disappear when I'm held accountable and when I'm looking forward to something. Getting fit with a friend is not only super fun but a great tool to push yourself to that next level. Share the love, share the sweat!"

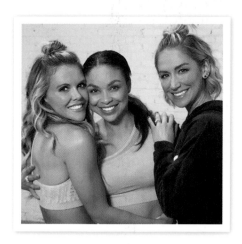

Chevy

Chevy, yoga sculpt trainer
for Studio Tone It Up,
@studiotoneitupchevy

"I love to look through and comment on #TIUteam photos on Insta-gram, and chat with the other girls in Studio Tone It Up before class. I'm also a big fan of making a *bomb* playlist that will inspire me during my workouts. And I'm a huge fan of mantras and affirmations. The words that I think about and use for motivation during workouts change often, but right now I'm really loving the word 'yes.' It's amazing what you can accomplish if instead of telling yourself 'No, I can't' or 'I won't,' you tell yourself 'Yes, I can, I will.'"

Jillian

Jillian, dance cardio trainer
for Studio Tone It Up,
@studiotoneitupjillian

"Music has to be my number one moti-vator. If I am by myself, it is headphones in and music turned up! Music can calm my mind by soothing it into a meditative yogic state, it can inspire me to create

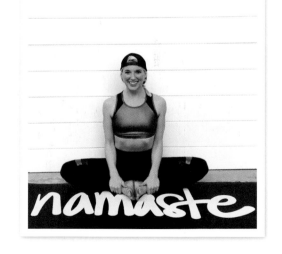

motivate

class choreography, it can pump me up and motivate me to push harder, and it can be an escape. I love creating playlists for my workouts and creating movement to match the music. Music can motivate me even when I am alone, but what really gives me that extra burst of motivation is community. The reason I got into the fitness industry is because I love sharing my passion for fitness with my community. There is nothing like a room full of women working out together, doing the same movements, at the same time, on the same musical beat. Those energetic vibrations set my soul on fire. The fact that a room full of people, from all walks of life, all on their own personal journey, can come together, work out together, and leave feeling better together is what really motivates me."

Chyna

Chyna, cardio kickboxing trainer
for Studio Tone It Up,
@studiotoneitupchyna

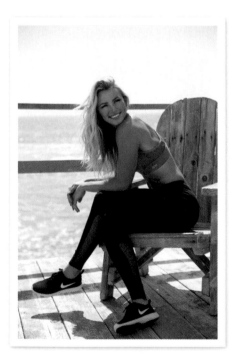

"I always say that the game changer for me was when I figured out my 'why.' Why am I working out? Is it to train for a half marathon? Is it to feel more confident and happy from the inside out? Is it to eventually be the best and healthiest mother I can be for my future children? Once you dig deep to find that 'why,' the drive will follow! The days you don't feel like working out, think about that 'why'!"

Tori

Tori, dance cardio trainer for
Studio Tone It Up, @studiotoneituptori

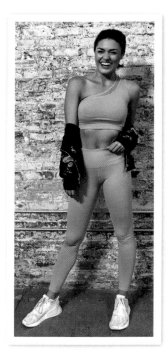

"When I want to give up or stop pushing, I simply re-member that I have a goal . . . but even more than that, I have a *plan* on how I'm going to reach that goal. I know that putting in the work is what makes reaching your goals so completely and utterly worth it. On days that I feel down, I turn to the people who support my goals—my family, my boyfriend, my accountability part-ner, my #TIUcommunity—and let them give me the extra push and words of encouragement that I need to fuel me to keep working toward my goals!"

Kristina

Kristina, cardio kickboxing and HIIT trainer
for Studio Tone It Up, @studiotoneitupkristina

"When I need a little extra motivation to exercise, I think of how far I've come. I was diagnosed with a heart condition when I was eight years old. In grade school, the nurses knew my name because I was con-stantly on their radar as the 'girl with fainting episodes.' When teachers or coaches would call an ambulance, I would cry because I didn't want to go to the hospital. Not because I was scared but because I simply wanted to be *normal*. I did not want the burden of always having to watch to make sure I did not overextend myself. It took about fifteen years for me, my family, and a team of doctors to get me to where I am

motivate

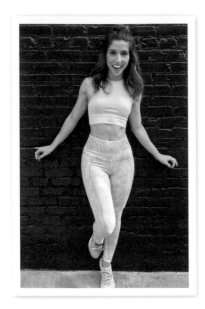

today. Once I felt strong enough, I started walk-jogging—mainly because my boyfriend (now husband!) was traveling a lot for work, and I needed a hobby. Those little walk-jogs turned into two triathlons, fourteen half marathons, two full marathons, and countless other races!

"So when I need that burst of motivation, I think back to the eight-year-old girl who couldn't complete a mile. I remember her, I *am* her, and today I will do everything in my power to prove to her that she is *strong*."

Sage

Sage Erickson, World Championship Tour surfer and Tone It Up athlete, @sageerickson

"If you need motivation to go for a new goal or reach for a new dream, remember you are always going to be a beginner at something! I wasn't always so great at surfing. It has taken time, passion, dedication, and a whole lot of losses. If you have an interest and put your mind to it, you will see the best

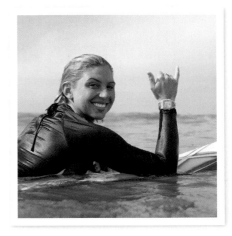

results! Remember, the experiences we have shape us into who we are. So choose things that mold you into someone you'd love to be around, because at the end of the day your happiness matters and it will be contagious to the ones you love around you!"

ACTION GUIDE
to Motivate

KATRINA It's time to take action! Karena and I asked our girls to share some of the most motivating times of their lives, when they felt powerful and fierce, and they shared tips that have helped them:

- Set a goal with an end date—something short-term that you can look forward to. Whether it's a beach trip, a festival, your birthday, a race, a date, graduation, spring break, a family vaca, or simply the start of summer so you can feel confident and healthy—anything that you can look forward to. You can book a mini photo shoot with your friends too. This is always fun to do so you can frame the pics after.

- Plan your entire week of workouts on the Sunday beforehand.

- It's super motivating to see results, so take before and after pics. Remember, the only time you look back is to see how far you've come.

- HIIT workouts are motivating! So is Tabata training, which is timed HIIT and you count how many reps you can do. We have Tabata workouts in the studio.

- Set up at least two workout dates per week.

- Commit to a Studio Tone It Up class with a friend. Did you know you can invite girlfriends within our app to work out with you? Karena and I will actually send you and your friend a notification reminding you of the class. It's really cool to be able to have accountability at your fingertips!

motivate

- Prep meals and enjoy mimosas together! (See our Rosé Mimosas recipe, page 113.) Get together on a Sunday (or on FaceTime) while you prep breakfasts, salads, snacks, and lean dinners for the week. It's a great way to make meal prep fun and productive.

- Even when you're working out or on a run, set yourself a goal to hit a certain number of minutes, or to keep going until you get to that street, or to reach a certain number of steps.

- Celebrate each milestone along your journey. Reward yourself with things that help you toward your goals, like a pass to more classes at your studio, a new yoga mat, or a massage.

Evening Tips

KARENA Kat and I love to plan ahead. One of the best habits we have is we set out our workout clothes each night for the next day. When we know it's going to be a busy week, we set out five outfits so we can grab 'n' go every morning. This is part of setting yourself up for success! I love to set out everything—even down to my socks and hair tie—so I'm not scrambling in the morning.

- Can't stop thinking about tomorrow? Us too! It helps to write on your to-do list anything that's on your mind. This way your mind will be at ease and you know you won't forget.

- Dear Diary . . . It's the perfect time to journal. We love to take note of things we want to remember from that day. Jot down your workouts, meals, and how you feel. It's important to look back and see when you tend to feel your best.

• Now it's time for your mini motivation mantra. You can either journal it or just think it to yourself before you fall asleep. You can say anything you like. It can be as simple as "I know I can do this" or "I'm beautiful, strong, and powerful" or "I can do anything I set my mind to."

 One mantra I love is from Deepak Chopra: "A miracle is a shift in perception from fear to love." Say that five times slowly . . . and tell us you don't feel at ease!

motivate

GET MOTIVATED
TO TAKE A RISK
AND CHASE
YOUR DREAMS

KATRINA Karena and I hear this question all the time: "What is your best advice for girls who want to change careers or follow their dreams?" We love helping other women go for something they're passionate about.

Our advice: It takes motivation, perseverance, and belief in yourself. And guess what—you have all those things! So just go for it. It's going to be scary, but where there's a will there's a way. We were so scared when we started Tone It Up—actually, we're still scared every day—but we know in our hearts that this is what we were meant to do, and everything is worth the sacrifice and hard work. If you're not a little scared, and your heart doesn't beat out of your chest thinking about the goal you want to achieve, we challenge you to dream bigger! You deserve to achieve the big dreams. There's so much you can accomplish, we promise you that. We hope that you believe in yourself, because we sure do.

- Close your eyes and see yourself achieving your goals. How do you feel? Confident? Fulfilled? Successful?

- How will you get there? Write down three short-term goals that will help you achieve your ultimate dream, and make a game plan for how and when you can put these goals into action. For example, if you want to get into fitness professionally, maybe your first goal is to take yoga teacher training, and you will look up the next one being offered in your area. When Karena and I signed up for our yoga training, we were both so nervous and excited. Do something that ignites you!

- Who can help you achieve it? Think about who can support you in your goal. Our husbands and each other were huge support systems when we went on tour and during our yoga teacher training. And we lean on each other and the Tone It Up community every day. Everyone needs support to make their dreams come true, so think about who in your family, friend group, and community will be the best support system for you. Then sit down with them and tell them about your goals and discuss how you can make them happen together.

- "If not now, when?" When we first heard this quote, it really resonated with us. As women, we put everything besides ourselves first. So if you're thinking of doing that something you've been waiting to do . . . get after it, girl! Don't wait for the right time—make the time! You'll be so grateful that you did.

motivate

What If My Motivation Dips?

KARENA   I dip, you dip, we dip! It's true—we all have times in our lives when we have a dip in motivation. Kat and I both have points when we're working crazy hours or we're feeling unmotivated and we stop focusing on our body, mind, and spirit. We forget to put ourselves first: we don't get enough sleep, we don't eat the best foods, we skip workouts, we aren't meditating, and we aren't connected to ourselves. But the best part is, you're just one workout away from a great mood. It really takes just one workout to be back at it. Whatever plateau or obstacle may be standing in your way, you'll bounce back even stronger. We know because we've been there too.

Here are our best tips for when your motivation dips:

- The most important thing is to always be kind to yourself. This is our top piece of advice. You are strong and beautiful. *Never* forget that, and always have compassion for yourself!

- Consistency is key. Make working out part of your lifestyle by making it a habit. Choose the best time of day to work out, and stick to it. We like to work out in the morning because it's before the crazy day begins and before other things can pop up and take priority.

- Don't give up if you're feeling stuck.

- Find new heights. Push yourself out of your comfort zone. You'll be amazed at what you find there. If you're always comfortable, you'll just sustain and maintain. And you deserve so much more! If you already work out consistently, mix it up with heavier weights, try out a new class in Studio Tone It Up

(Dance cardio anyone? Or HIIT?), or take your workouts outside. Mixing it up will rev up your metabolism and keep your body guessing. Just continue to work out regularly.

- Keeping a food journal is an excellent tool for tracking what you eat and drink. It's hard to remember everything without writing it down. Be sure to take note if there are certain times during the day, or certain days, when you have specific cravings. Time to refocus on "lean, clean, 'n' green" on Fridays and Saturdays. With a little wine and chocolate mixed in too!

- Lean on your team. Don't be afraid to be vulnerable. Reach out to your friends and tell them what's going on. They're there for you.

- Treat yo'self, girl! You deserve some R and R and pampering. This means making the time to do the things you love and that are nourishing for your mind, body, and spirit. Maybe it's a mani or taking a long bubble bath with some Epsom salt and essential oils. Or head to a new workout studio you've been wanting to try. Whatever it is, we want you to feel like a freaking goddess after!

motivate

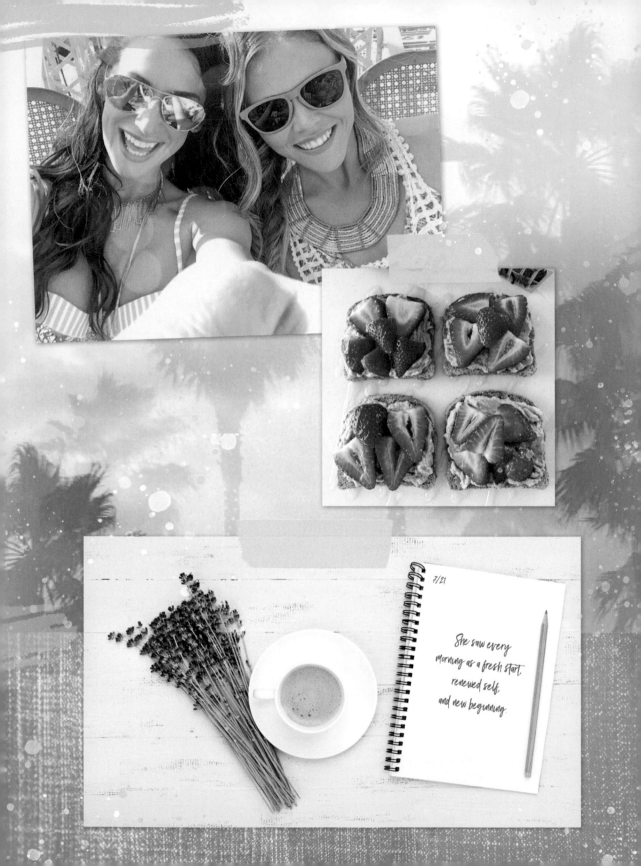

7/21

She saw every
morning as a fresh start,
renewed self,
and new beginning.

Vision Board to Motivate

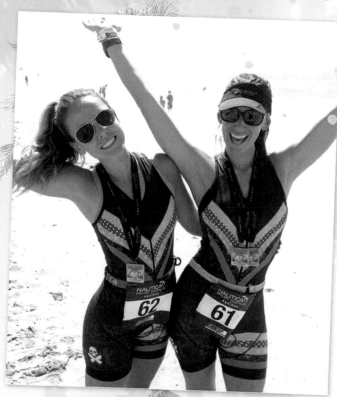

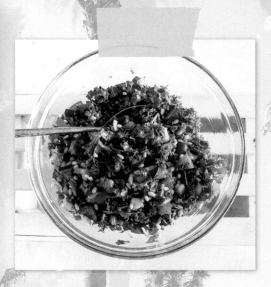

REFLECT
to Motivate

I felt most motivated today when

_____

A new thing I can do to feel motivated is

_____

My role model when it comes to motivation is

_____

A fitness goal that will motivate me is

_____

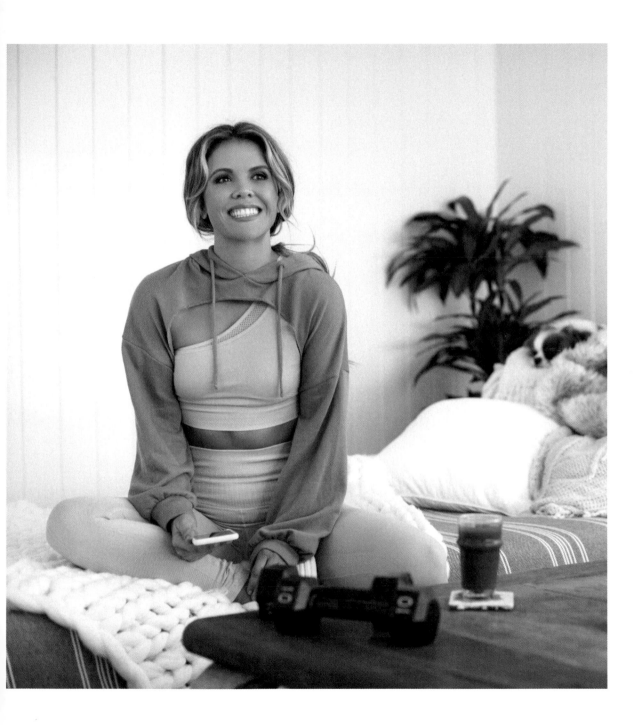

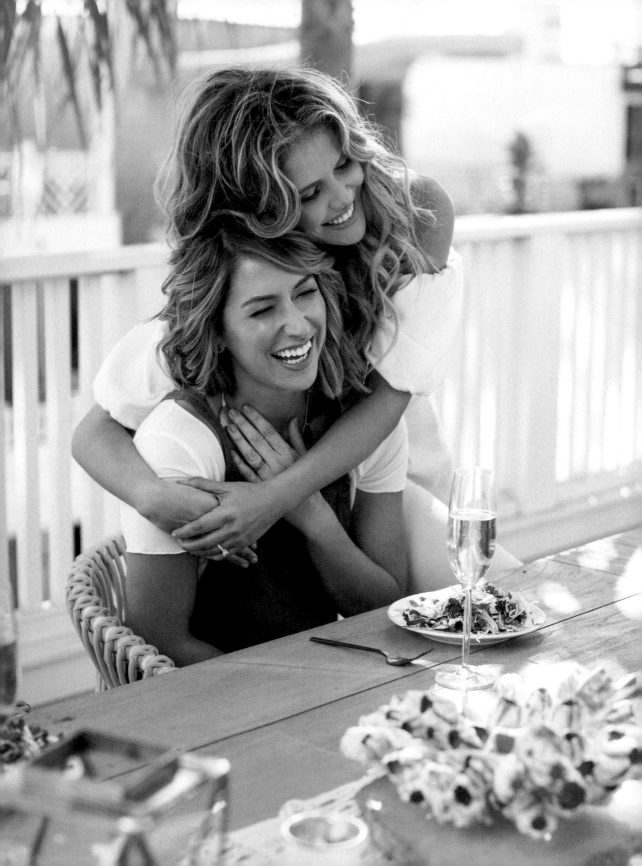

3

Inspire

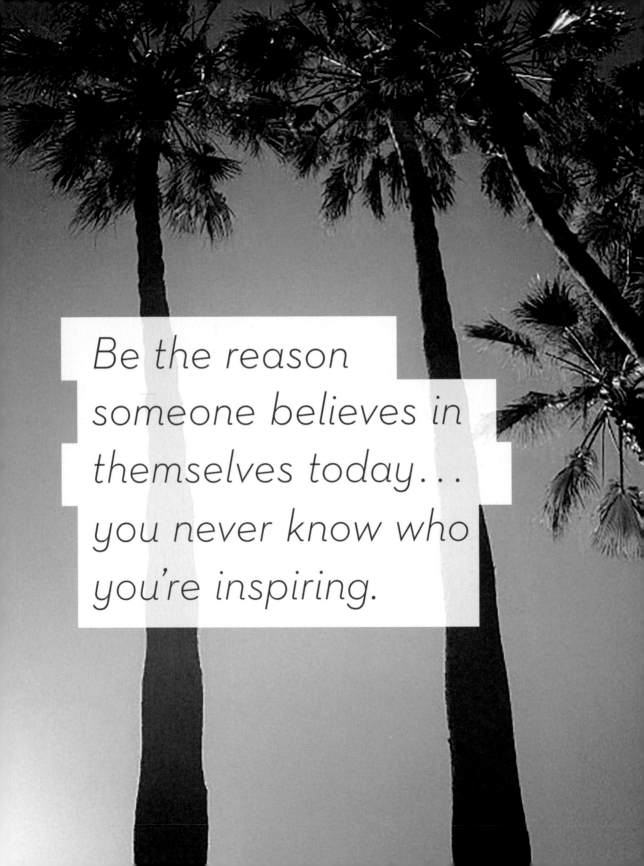

Be the reason someone believes in themselves today... you never know who you're inspiring.

GIRL TALK
to Inspire

KARENA This chapter struck home for me. I really had to sit back and think about what inspiration truly is. It's different from motivation, or feeling energized. What I realized is that sometimes inspirational moments come when we're not motivated or don't have the energy to move forward but we push through anyway. Some of the most inspirational stories we hear or watch online, on TV, or on the news are about people who achieve greatness and love under some of the most difficult circumstances.

Like I mentioned in my story, I felt the most inspired in my life when I turned it around from a dark place and was brave enough to change, dig deep within, reconnect with my body, and awaken my entire soul. When I started to compete in triathlons, my healing began. I can remember looking at how I turned my life around and thinking, *Well, if I can do it, then truly anyone can.* Within the past year, I've endured some difficult times with my mom and her health. Physical and mental illness affects not only the diagnosed but everyone around them too. This year, I'm inspired by my ability, through exhaustion and pure frustration, to become a caretaker for someone who didn't want to be saved and didn't want to fight for her own life. I did what I knew I had to do; I fought for her, and I've fought hard.

As life untangles and obstacles arise, you uncover things about yourself that you never knew you had inside—your growth, your patience, your truth. Through pain, you learn a lot. And as painful as

inspire

something may be, sometimes it's inspiring to be able to shift your perspective, which makes you stronger. I'm now more inspired than ever to take better care of myself—mindfully, physically, and spiritually. It also inspired me to join NAMI, the National Alliance on Mental Illness, where I'm learning how to better understand and have empathy for those with mental illness and receive crisis education. I hope to use what I've learned to support and inspire others who may be in similar situations.

So when it comes to you and your inspiration, think about all you have overcome and all you are capable of. I'm already inspired by you for taking this step. Reach out for support from people in your life who inspire you too. For my own inspiration and support, I've always looked to my father, who has been through hard times and darkness in our family. He found peace and love again. I also look to Bobby—he's my foundation and my rock. And I look to Kat, who inspires me with her endless love, care, and compassion. I confide in my yoga and spiritual teachers too, to connect with enlightenment.

Think about what inspires you. Is it your strength to overcome? Is it a special person, a book, or a quote? The best thing about inspiration is that it can come from anywhere, from anyone, and at any time. And it will help you achieve all your dreams and discover new ones beyond what you ever thought possible!

SPIRITUAL GUIDE
to Inspire

KATRINA   Devote your morning to you. Karena and I know the mornings can be hectic, between running out the door to get to work, maybe getting your family ready for school, and all your other obligations and to-do lists. We completely understand. What if you woke up a little earlier, before anyone else, and devoted the first part of your morning to you? What if you took time for yourself? How much more energized, balanced, relaxed, and inspired would you feel?

You deserve this time. You may need to get to bed a little earlier to make this happen, but we promise it will be so worth it. When you put yourself first, you are able to be a better coworker, partner, parent, and friend all day long.

What Inspires Me

I find inspiration in perseverance. Life will no doubt try to knock you down and drag you backward. When I see others take their struggles and turn them into strengths to follow their dreams, it inspires me even more to discover what life is trying to teach me and to always move forward.

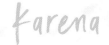

What Inspires Me

What inspires me most is seeing women reach their full potential. Nothing makes me happier or more inspired than knowing that the women in my life and in the Tone It Up community are thriving, ignited, fulfilled, and feeling like their absolute strongest and most beautiful selves. It's pretty powerful.

Katrina

inspire

CREATE AN INSPIRATION AREA IN YOUR HOME

KARENA I love and cherish my mornings. I wake up early before my husband, Bobby, and go upstairs. I light a fire in the fireplace and all my favorite scented candles and take a few minutes to meditate and give gratitude, read a passage from one of my favorite inspirational books (see my picks on page 193), and set my intentions for the day. Or I head to my small meditation room, which I've filled with candles, pillows, essential oils, and books. I even put up a chalkboard where I write my favorite inspirational quotes. I love walking into this room, as it is so full of positive energy. So even if I have only five minutes before Bobby wakes up and I have to get myself out the door, I try to spend time every morning in either the living room or my meditation room. On weekends when I have more time, I aim for at least thirty minutes of me time. This always helps center and inspire me for the day. When I feel ready, I let the rest of the world back in and get to work.

To create your own meditation or inspiration space, you don't need an entire room or anything big. All it takes is a nook in your living room or bedroom. Here are some ideas to prepare your own space:

- Add scented candles or a diffuser with fragrant essential oils. I also burn sage (which is very purifying) or palo santo (which means "holy wood"—it comes from a tree grown in South America, is also purifying, and smells divine, like a combination of citrus, mint, and pine).

- Print out some of your favorite photos of friends or family who inspire you, and create a picture wall. Or frame some of your favorite inspirational quotes to hang on the wall.

- Bring in your phone with a playlist of inspiring music. Whatever moves you—it's different for everyone. And you can switch this up every day, depending on your mood.

- Have a bottle of cold water, a cup of hot tea, or your morning coffee at hand in case you get thirsty. You can even try drinking a certain kind of tea or other drink daily in your special space so your brain will quickly associate the aroma and taste with your meditation and inspiration.

- Go ahead and hold on to objects or souvenirs with special meaning to you. For me, that's crystals. I just love them, because they represent the energy I need to surround myself with. Crystals come from the earth, so they are charged with energy the way all minerals are, and each kind of crystal has a special vibe to it. My favorites are amethyst (known for divine connection, healing properties, and calming qualities), black tourmaline (used for grounding and as protection against negative energy), citrine (known for promoting abundance, manifestation, creativity, and good fortune), rose quartz (known for opening the heart to giving and receiving love, emotional healing/calming, and providing relief after any kind of upset), selenite (known for spiritual activation, connecting with your higher self, clearing negative energy and improving your own energy, and clarity), and crystal quartz (known as the "master healer" and for amplifying the energy of all the other crystals you have as well as your intentions). Even if you don't believe in these kinds of attributes, every crystal is unique, and they're really beautiful objects to fill your inspiration space. Just looking at them makes you feel at ease.

inspire

We always find the most inspiration in the mornings. Our favorite way to start the day is by having a mindful morning. Light a candle, pour some coffee, sit in a peaceful space, breathe deeply, and take those few special minutes to connect with yourself. It's a perfect way to create space, be present, and set your intentions for the day. Is it gorgeous outside? Take your coffee on a little coffee walk for 10 to 15 minutes.

Start Each Day with Intention

There is *major* power in putting your intentions on paper! Writing down your goals in a journal is like making a promise to yourself, and that is the most important promise you can make. Start by taking five minutes each morning to journal your intentions, and before long it will be as natural as brushing your teeth or sipping your coffee.

Close your eyes and think about what you need for the day and what others in your life need from you. Are you feeling like you need to challenge yourself and say yes to a new adventure? Do you need to be kinder to yourself and show yourself grace? Does a friend or family member need a little extra love and support? Does a colleague need leadership? Let that guide your intentions. Doing this always makes us feel strong and prepared to handle anything that comes our way for the rest of the day.

K&K's Favorite Inspiring Yoga Mantras

To relieve stress, I do yoga . . .
Just kidding. I drink wine in my yoga pants.

—UNKNOWN

KARENA I recited the following mantra during our yoga practice on the Tone It Up Tour. It resonated with us and our community, so it holds a special place in my heart:

> May we loosen our grip and open our hearts.
>
> May we release all that is no longer a vibrational match.
>
> May our hearts be open, stretched, and full.
>
> May our arms and minds stay open so that what is on its way can arrive swiftly.
>
> May our mouths be used as vehicles of truth, integrity, and peace.
>
> May our creations travel, our new projects be ignited, our deepest prayers be heard, and our hearts held by the mysterious force that simply is.
>
> And so it is, and so it is, and so it is.
>
> —Rebecca Campbell,
> Rise Sister Rise

inspire

As an assignment for my yoga teacher training, I read the book *Journey into Power* by Baron Baptiste, an expert in power yoga. I love his perspective:

> When you hit your edge in a pose—or in your everyday life—instead of giving in to frustration or whatever other reaction surfaces, focus on your commitment to grow and ask yourself: Where am I now and can I accept, let go, and grow?
>
> —Baron Baptiste,
> *Journey into Power*

KATRINA

> The one thing that you have that nobody else has is you. Your voice, your mind, your story, your vision. So write and draw and build and play and dance and live only as you can.
>
> —Neil Gaiman,
> University of the Arts'
> commencement address

> Be a reflection of what you'd like to receive. If you want love, give love. If you want truth, be truthful. What you give out will always return.
>
> —Kristen Butler,
> Power of Positivity

> Participate relentlessly in the manifestation of your own blessings.
>
> —Elizabeth Gilbert,
> *Eat Pray Love*

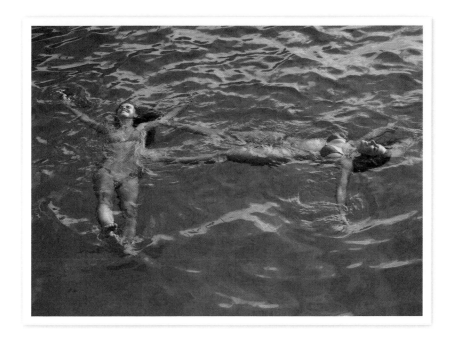

I wrote this during my yoga teacher training and read it to the Tone It Up community during my first live class:

> Your vibe is your most powerful quality. The vibe you bring is what you receive. What you need, you must give first. Your surroundings are completely up to you. How do you show up? How do you present your most authentic self? Your vibe attracts your tribe . . . and your best life.

I also love this mantra from my absolute fave human in the world:

> Quiet the mind and bring your intention inward. When we give ourselves that personal silence, we often find what we are looking for.
>
> —Karena Dawn

WORKOUT GUIDE
to Inspire

All right, babe, you ready? We want you to do as many of these moves as you can today.

Exercises for Your Booty . . . Because Your Booty Inspires Us!

Here again you may start these exercises with a heavier set of weights—12 to 15 pounds—and complete as many reps as you can with proper form, then drop down to a lower weight.

Do *three circuits* of the following:

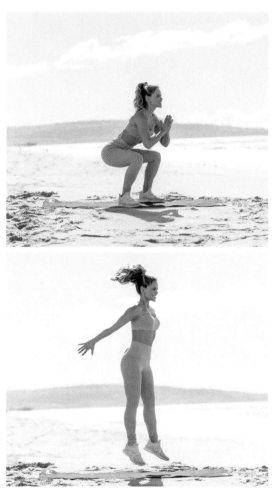

1 Squat Jump Challenge

10 SQUATS, 10 SQUAT JUMPS,
9 SQUATS, 9 SQUAT JUMPS . . .
COUNTING DOWN TO 1.

2 Dead Lift

15 REPS (YOUR BOOTY IS STRONG!
START WITH THE HEAVIER SET
OF WEIGHTS FOR THIS MOVE.)

inspire

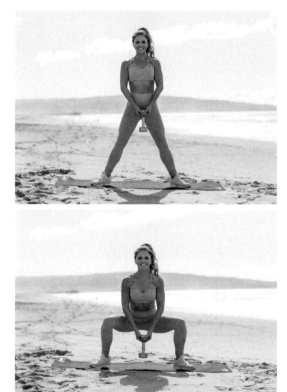

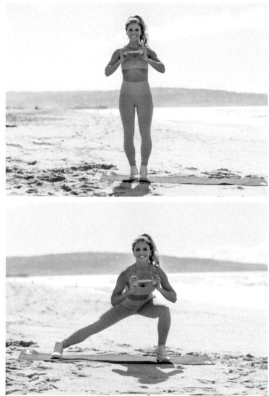

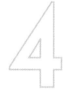 *Sumo Squat*

15 REPS

4 *Weighted Side Lunge*

15 REPS ON EACH SIDE

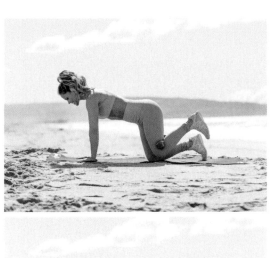

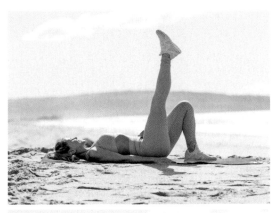

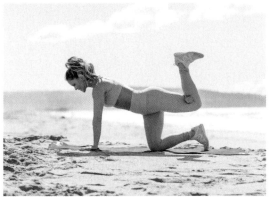

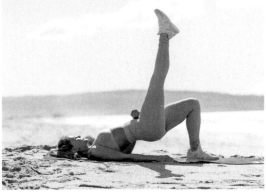

5 *Weighted Donkey Kick*

15 REPS ON EACH SIDE

6 *Weighted Single Leg Bridge*

15 REPS ON EACH SIDE

inspire

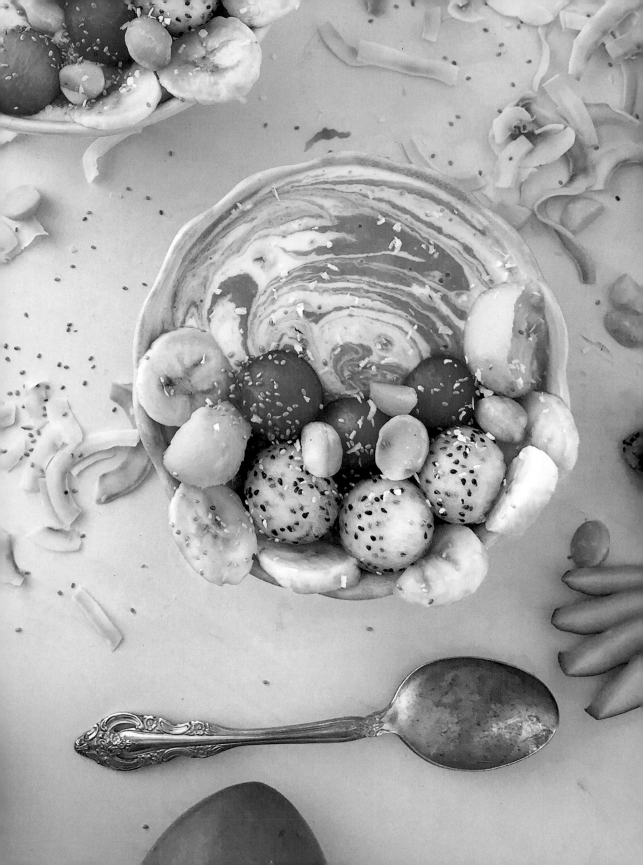

RECIPE GUIDE
to Inspire

TROPICAL PARADISE
SMOOTHIE BOWL

Serves 1

½ cup coconut water

1 scoop coconut
Tone It Up Protein

¼ cup chopped
frozen mango

½ frozen banana

¼ cup chopped
frozen papaya

1 tablespoon
macadamia nuts

Toppings (optional):
Swirl of coconut
cream, 1 tablespoon
unsweetened coconut
flakes, 2 teaspoons
chia seeds, 2 teaspoons
cacao nibs, or your
favorite fruit

In a high-speed blender, puree the coconut water, Tone It Up Protein,
mango, banana, papaya, and macadamia nuts until the mixture is smooth.

Serve with a combination of two or three toppings, if you like.

inspire

LOVE YOU SO
MATCHA DONUTS

Makes 4 (1 donut per serving)

½ cup oat flour

½ cup vanilla Tone It Up Protein

1 teaspoon baking powder

½ teaspoon ground cinnamon

Pinch of salt

1 egg

¼ cup unsweetened almond milk

¼ cup maple syrup

1 teaspoon vanilla extract

1 tablespoon melted coconut oil

Coconut oil spray

FOR THE GLAZE

1 cup unsweetened almond milk or coconut milk yogurt

1 teaspoon matcha

Preheat the oven to 350°F.

In a mixing bowl, combine the oat flour, Tone It Up Protein, baking powder, cinnamon, and salt.

In a separate bowl, whisk together the egg, almond milk, maple syrup, vanilla extract, and melted coconut oil.

Add the wet ingredients to the dry, and stir to combine the mixture well.

Coat a donut pan with coconut oil spray, and spoon in the batter to make 4 donuts. Bake them for 15 to 20 minutes, or until a toothpick comes out clean.

As the donuts are baking, you can make the glaze by whisking together the glaze ingredients in a small bowl. When the donuts are slightly cooled, dip them in the glaze or drizzle the glaze over them.

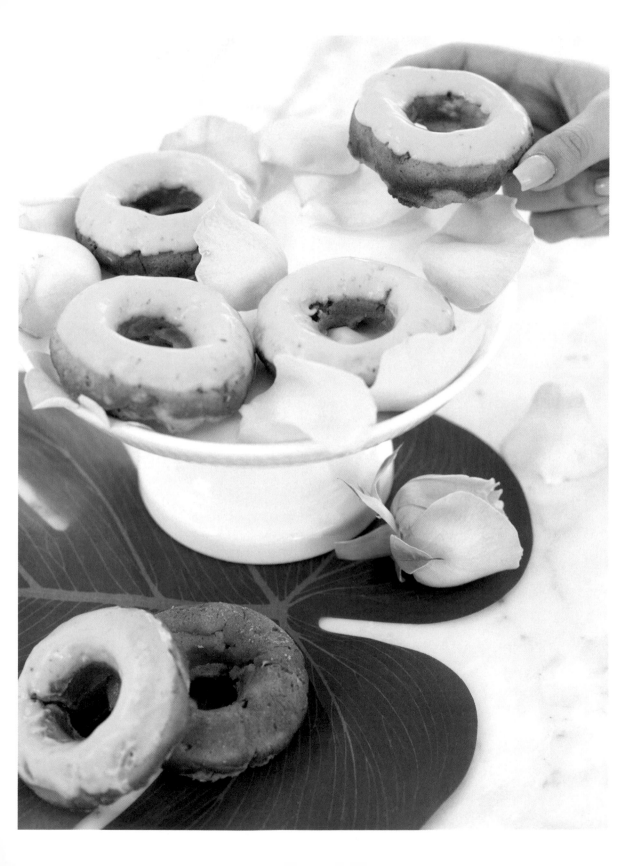

TURQUOISE BOWL

Serves 1

If we could have this every day, we would! It's so delicious, and it's packed with protein, iron, calcium, vitamins A, B, and E, and healthy fats. It's also extremely anti-inflammatory and filled with antioxidants.

½ frozen banana

1 date, pitted

1 teaspoon maca powder

2 tablespoons slivered almonds

2 teaspoons chia seeds

1 tablespoon unsweetened cocoa powder

½ teaspoon spirulina

1 scoop vanilla Tone It Up Protein

½ teaspoon ground cinnamon

1 cup coconut water

½ cup ice

Cacao nibs (optional)

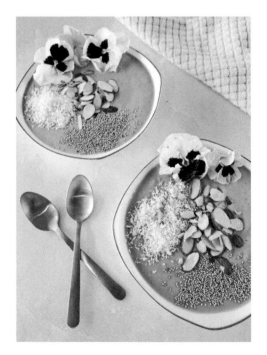

In a high-speed blender, puree the banana, date, maca, almonds, chia seeds, cocoa powder, spirulina, Tone It Up Protein, cinnamon, and coconut water until the mixture is smooth.

Add the ice and blend on a high setting until it's creamy.

Serve topped with a sprinkle of cacao nibs, if desired. Garnish with edible flowers.

ROSÉ MIMOSAS

Simply combine sparkling rosé with grapefruit juice!

PINK LATTE

Serves 1

1 small beet, peeled

1 cup unsweetened almond milk

1 teaspoon honey

½ teaspoon ground cinnamon

¼ teaspoon ginger powder

Preheat the oven to 425°F.

Wrap the beet in foil and pierce the foil with a fork. Bake it for 20 to 30 minutes.

When the beet is cooked all the way through, put it in a blender with the almond milk, honey, cinnamon, and ginger, and blend until the mixture is smooth.

Strain the liquid through a strainer or cheesecloth, then heat it in a pot set over medium heat.

Pour the hot latte into a cup, and sprinkle it with a dash more cinnamon. You can also add some edible flowers on top. Enjoy!

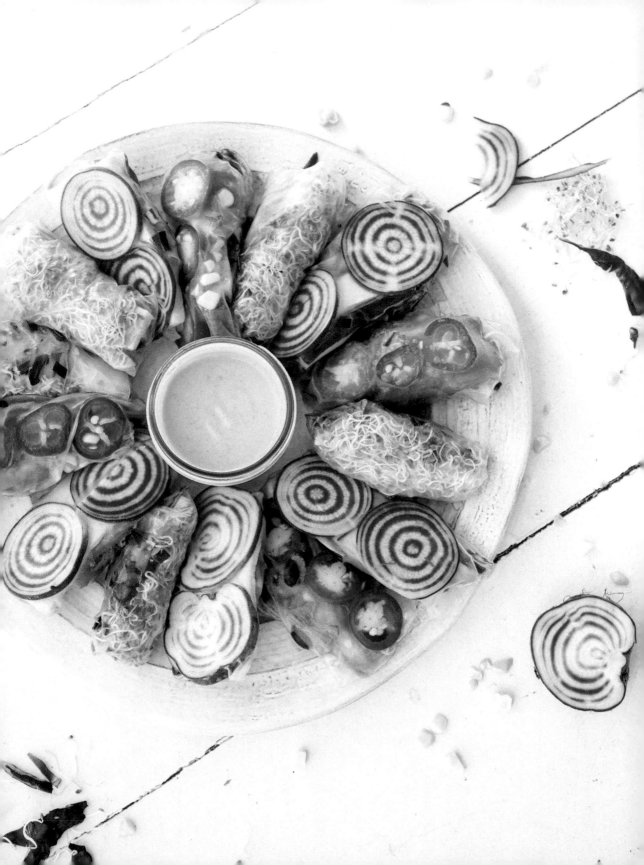

SEXY SPRING ROLLS
with MISO DRESSING

Makes 3 (1 serving)

3 sheets square
spring roll rice paper

1 cup bean sprouts

1/2 medium raw beet,
sliced

1/2 medium raw zucchini
sliced

1 jalapeño, thinly sliced

6 ounces lean protein

3 slices peeled and
pitted avocado

3 tablespoons minced
fresh parsley

FOR THE DRESSING

1 tablespoon white
or yellow miso

Juice of 1 lemon

1 tablespoon water

Soak each sheet of rice paper in water until it is soft. Lay one out on a flat surface.

Add one-third quantity of the bean sprouts, beet, zucchini, jalapeño, protein, avocado, and parsley to the center of the paper while leaving about an inch or more on all sides. Tuck in the top and bottom edges, then roll one side over and keep rolling until it forms a burrito shape. Repeat this for the other two rolls. Set the rolls on a plate.

In a small bowl, combine the dressing ingredients with a fork, and enjoy it as a dip for the rolls.

inspire

SUNDAYS ARE FOR SUNDAES

Serves 3

1 1/2 cups diced
frozen banana

1/4 cup dairy-free milk
(almond, coconut, cashew,
hemp seed, hazelnut, oat)

Pinch of Himalayan sea salt

FLAVOR CHOICES

Vanilla: 1/2 tablespoon
maple syrup and 1 teaspoon
vanilla extract or fresh
vanilla bean seeds

Chocolate: 1 tablespoon
maple syrup and
1 tablespoon unsweetened
cocoa powder

Pistachio: 1 tablespoon
maple syrup and 1/4 cup
chopped pistachios

Strawberry: 1/2 tablespoon
maple syrup and 1/4 cup
sliced fresh strawberries

Coconut: 1 tablespoon
maple syrup and 1/4 cup
unsweetened shredded
coconut

TOPPINGS

Cacao nibs or
dark chocolate

Almond slivers

Unsweetened
coconut flakes

Dried goji berries

Fresh berries

Gluten-free granola

In a high-speed blender, puree all the ingredients for the base of the sundaes with a flavor of your choice. You may have to stop and push the mixture down every 30 seconds or so to reach a smooth consistency.

Serve the sundaes with dishes offering each of our fave toppings listed.

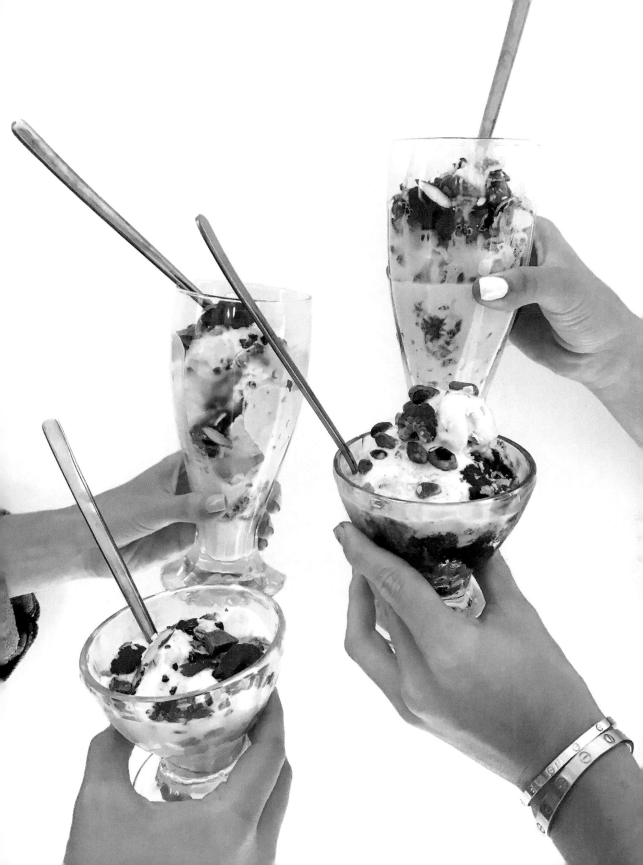

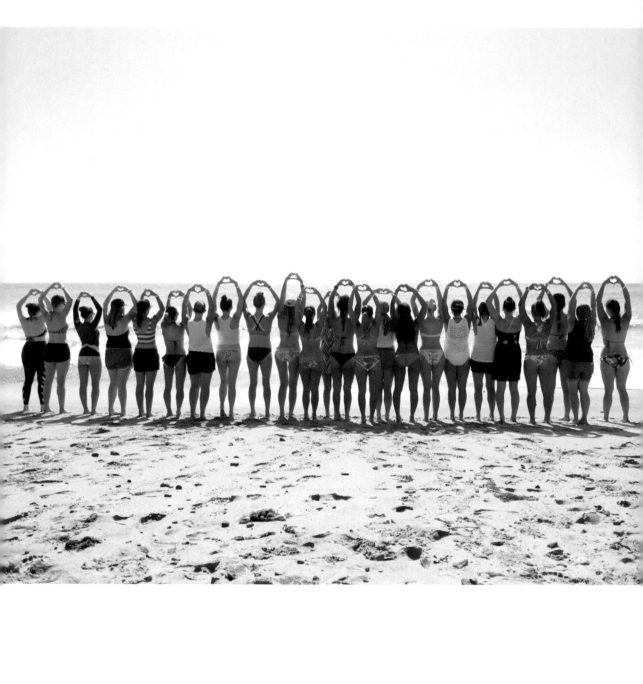

GIRLFRIEND GUIDE
to Inspire

KATRINA I believe it takes being an amazing friend to have amazing friends. It's so important to make time for others—to listen and be there for them. In turn, you'll have really strong female relationships in your life. Karena and I have a strong friendship because we are always there for each other. Whatever you feel you need in your life, give that first, and it will come back around.

I'm also so grateful to have my close girlfriends of more than sixteen years. They're like sisters to me. It wasn't always easy, though. At one point we all lived in different cities and could connect only by phone or FaceTime, but we made the effort to not only call each other but also book trips to see each other. We would drop everything to either visit for a weekend or travel to a new place for a girls' getaway. I'm so happy we started that tradition, because now, years later, we all live close to one another in California. The strong bond we have and the little things we did to keep our friendships alive led us all to this place together. There truly are no coincidences in life, just the magic of love.

It's so important to make your female relationships a priority in your life, because you never know when you'll need each other or a little inspiration.

Inspirational Get-Togethers

KATRINA Karena and I texted our friends and asked what inspires them when we all get together, and everyone across the board said "Discovering something new" or "Setting up something beautiful together."

We're always on the lookout for local events. We actually have an app that shows local concerts—singer-songwriters, indie musicians, or big bands coming to town. It also alerts us to museum events, art shows, outdoor movie screenings, restaurant openings, plays, street festivals, and even flea markets. If you search locally, you too can probably find a source that gives you the heads-up in your town. We find inspiration in experiencing new things together, especially art and history.

Here are some tips for throwing a mini inspo celebration:

- Take a hike! No, but seriously—hike. Karena and I went hiking on my birthday, and we made it to the top of the trail for the sunrise over the mountains in Malibu! It was really inspiring and motivating.

- Host a babe brunch! Invite your girls over for Tone It Up Pancakes (page 201) and Rosé Mimosas (page 113). Set up an inspiring table by including quotes at each place setting.

- At one of our get-togethers, we brought out all our large pillows and poufs instead of chairs—think boho chic.

- Mismatched pillows and low crates as coffee tables look amazing together.

- String bistro lights or mini twinkle lights, and use votives and tea lights on the table. Reuse votives forever—they go a long way toward making your table look gorgeous. I picked up pink Depression-style glass votives and vases at a flea market, and I've been using them for years!

PICNIC THREE BEAN SALAD

Serves 2

This salad is really flavorful and filling, and super easy to make.
Karena's been making it for our picnics and barbecues
for years, and it's always a hit.

½ cup canned cannellini
beans, drained and rinsed

½ cup canned chickpeas,
drained and rinsed

½ cup canned kidney
beans, drained and rinsed

¼ cup chopped celery

2 tablespoons chopped
red onions

2 tablespoons chopped
fresh cilantro

2 tablespoons chopped
fresh rosemary

2 tablespoons apple cider
vinegar

2 tablespoons olive oil

Pinch of salt and pepper

In a bowl, toss together all the
ingredients, and it's ready to go!

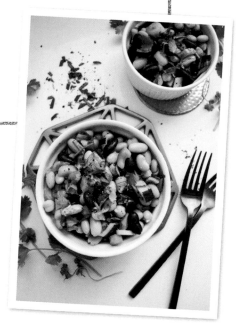

inspire

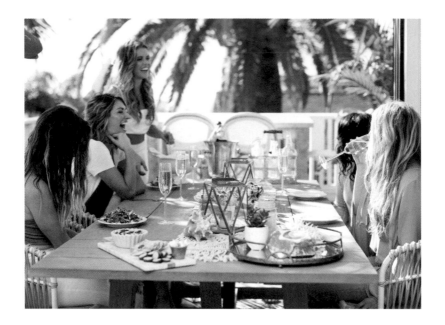

- Bring a projector for a movie night in the park or a slideshow to surprise your girls with old pics throughout the years. I did this for a friend's engagement party, and it was a huge hit!

- Make inspiration boards together: everyone brings magazines, quotes, inspiring images, medals from races, and anything they want to add to their board.

- Keep the menu simple. We love to make up large platters with vibrant veggies, like red and green peppers, broccoli, cherry tomatoes, purple cauliflower, carrots, cucumbers, and rainbow radishes. Serve the veggies with a hummus or spinach dip. Check out our favorite party dips (guacamole recipes on pages 157 and 161). We also make a large fruit platter with berries, grapes, watermelon, mango, and grapefruit.

- Don't forget to give a host toast! Toast your girlfriends and share why they inspire you.

BEAUTY TIPS
to Inspire

- We love wearing inspiring tanks while we work out. We have some on ToneItUp.com. The latest is "No pain, no champagne"—there's some real inspo!

- Watch beauty tutorials on YouTube for new ideas.

- Look up fun ways to mix up your eye makeup, like bright eyeliner.

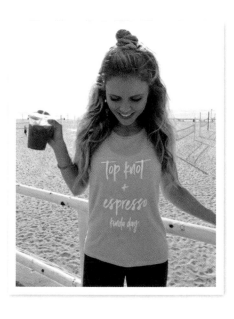

- Vintage clothes shopping can inspire you with ideas from different eras to help you step out of your comfort zone. This is one of Karena's fave things to do!

- Thrifting is inspiring— exploring old and new beauty.

inspire

CONNECT WITH THE TONE IT UP COMMUNITY
to Inspire

We are constantly inspired by the strong, brilliant, and gorgeous women of the Tone It Up community. We all come from different backgrounds and have unique voices, and we all are striving together to uplift each other and make each other stronger. Meet some of the inspiring women of the Tone It Up team, and read their incredible stories.

Stories from Community Members

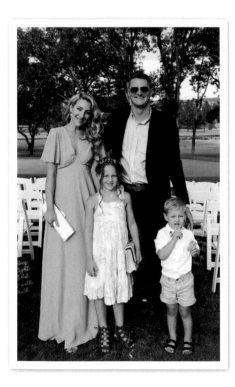

Naomi and family

Naomi @naomitonesitup

"Hi, I'm Naomi! I'm a wife and mama of two. I grew up active and played sports most of my life. Working out was something that I did most of my adult life, and I never really struggled with losing weight until I had my second child. I felt stuck with 30 extra pounds that just wouldn't leave. I tried every fad diet out there, but it wasn't until I started my Tone It Up journey in April 2017 that I had success.

"The Tone It Up lifestyle *changed my life*! I have lost 30 pounds since then, but more importantly I have changed the way I view myself and my body. For the first time in my life, I've learned to love my body! I have found this amazing community of like-minded and positive women to check in with and who are there for me every single day!

"In December of 2017, my 'healthy' thirty-three-year-old husband suffered four heart attacks in less than twenty-four hours, and he was hospitalized for six days in the Critical Care Unit. It was the scariest time of life! I still get teary-eyed when I think about the love and support I received through the TIU community. I had thousands of messages from girls in the community, flowers, notes, and gifts sent to me from all over the world! It was truly humbling and I never felt alone. This community lifted my spirits when I needed it the most and gave me hope that my husband was going to be okay. For that, I am forever grateful to this community and proud to be a TIU girl!

"My husband's heart issues are still unknown, but I'm happy to report he is on the road to recovery. He does have limitations on what he can do, but we are taking it one day at a time. I see my husband's health limitations and I find inspiration to push myself to new levels of fitness and become stronger—because I am able! In life, there will always be obstacles and struggles, but I firmly believe if you stay positive and strong during those hardships you will get through anything life throws at you. I'm so beyond grateful for life, my health, my strong body, and the constant love and support from the amazing TIU community."

inspire

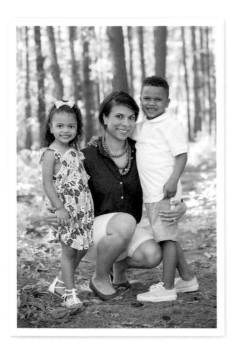

Joy and family

Joy @tiu_joystl

"I'm a thirty-six-year-old wife, mother of two, and business owner. I love fitness and nutrition, laughing, a great movie, shopping, and ice cream!

"In the summer of 2017, I joined the Tone It Up Eight-Week Bikini Series. When we began the Bikini Series, I was almost two months pregnant with my third child. By the end of week two, I was going strong on nutrition and consistent with my workouts but started feeling 'not right.' In the middle of doing a yoga workout I had to stop because I was experiencing pain. By that night, I was in the ER and I was in danger of having a miscarriage. I stayed at home that weekend. Of course I stopped working out, in fear of losing the baby and out of sheer necessity due to the pain I was in. My symptoms unfortunately just revved up from there. The following week, I miscarried. I was emotionally distraught, tired, discouraged, and unmotivated. I was just numb. I didn't know what to do.

"That is until Wednesday, May 3rd, when @sarahjett_tiu, the beautiful girl who helped turn my world around, reached out to me. I didn't know her. We had never spoken, only followed each other in the Tone It Up Instagram community. She said these simple words: 'Hey, girl! Haven't seen any posts from you in a while, so just thought I'd check in and see how everything's going?' I started crying and felt a surge of hope rise up in me that I can't explain. How can someone I don't even know make me feel this renewed sense of purpose again?

"I don't think you can even begin to realize just *how* much this community of women affects lives day in and day out. I had energy to focus on this challenge, and I gave it my all. Through the emotional and physical pain I endured, I had my TIU workouts to focus on, check-ins to look forward to, all the encouragement, the opportunity to encourage others as they pressed through their day to day. This will always be one of the most memorable of times for me, and I will look back fondly, because at the end of it all I gained strength and resilience. I pushed past the fear and pain. I'm grateful."

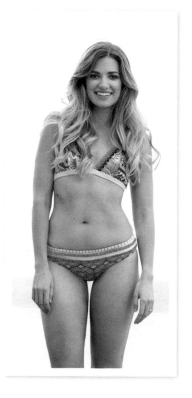

Yassi

Yassi @yassi_tiu

"I'm Yassi, a fitness-obsessed NYC local (beach babe at heart!) and coding nerd! I had a pretty unhealthy childhood, mostly stemming from my family's own struggles with health and fitness. Both of my parents were obese, as well as every other extended family member on both sides of my family. They all struggled with high blood pressure, diabetes, and eventually cancer, which ultimately caused my mother's passing when I was sixteen (she was only fifty). I was diagnosed with high blood pressure when I turned twenty, which was a giant defining moment in my journey. I was slightly overweight, but nothing too drastic, and with no other health symptoms. I started to wonder, *Is this how it starts? Is this the beginning of the slippery slope?* It became clear that if I was already starting to get sick at twenty, then I was already on the road to repeating my family's mistakes. That idea scared me more than anything. I made a promise with myself: continuing to live the life I had, with all of my habits, was no longer an option. That was such a wonderful moment, because I realized that I was willing to try (and possibly even fail) at anything on this journey, just as long as I wasn't back where I started.

"After finding Tone It Up, I became so excited to start my own journey. I went into the TIU community and found so many other women, just like me, who had the same goals and were also achieving results! Suddenly, the life that I was dreaming of wasn't so out of reach. Every day, I could talk to like-minded women about my struggles, heartbreaks, and triumphs. They all understood me and knew how difficult this journey would be. Having that support system and constant encouragement was so vital to my success, and I honestly don't think I would have been successful without all of the amazing women in this community who cheer each other on. Everyone believes in you here, and that helps you believe in yourself even more.

"One of the things that I learned with my journey through Tone It Up is to be honest with myself in regards to what makes me happy and what makes me feel good. I figured out what food and exercise plans made me feel the best, so why couldn't I take that mindset and apply that to my career? I realized that I deserved a career that made me leap out of bed in the morning and made me feel excited about what I do on a daily basis. I did some soul-searching and decided to go back to school and become a full-stack web developer! Starting Tone It Up taught me how to go out and create the life that I want and deserve."

ACTION GUIDE
to Inspire

It's evening and you're settling in. Now is the perfect time to reflect on your day.

Acknowledge Everything You Accomplished

It's just as important to revisit your intentions when the day is done as it is to set them in the morning.

Acknowledging everything you accomplished can be done as quietly as a meditation with yourself or journal writing, or by expressing it outwardly. Allow yourself to focus on gratitude again. Thank your body for all it does for you. Thank anyone who helped you during the day. Thank yourself for setting aside time to prioritize *you*. You did an amazing thing for yourself, and you deserve recognition.

- If you didn't quite meet all your goals and intentions, it's okay! Don't be hard on yourself. This happens to all of us. Be kind to yourself instead. Guilt doesn't serve you and can actually prevent you from reaching your goals. Don't sweat the small stuff. Instead, look forward to tomorrow and all the amazing things that are ahead of you.

Our Favorite Ways to Unwind

We know, we know . . . the latest episode on Netflix is calling your name. But we want you to go to sleep earlier than usual tonight. It will help you wake up earlier tomorrow to have that extra time for you. If you're doing something before bed, ask yourself, "Will this serve my goals in the morning?" Instagram-stalking your best friend's cousin's girlfriend definitely won't!

- At least an hour before bedtime put the electronics away. Turn the ringer off on your phone, and close your laptop. The blue light from the screens on electronics actually makes it hard for your busy brain to shut down and receive the signals that it's time for beauty sleep. Instead, add a soothing hot bath, a steaming cup of delicious chamomile tea, and a book to your nighttime routine. You'll thank us tomorrow when you feel beautiful and refreshed.

- Make the bed you sleep in . . . and make it amazing. Create a space that you look forward to jumping into after a long day. This is where you reenergize your body (aka your sanctuary). Think soft sheets, cozy blankets, the perfect pillow, and maybe even a silk pillowcase. You deserve to get your beauty z's.

- Cool it! Did you know that your body temperature drops when you go to sleep? A cool room tells your brain to get ready to dream. Crack open a window and get a fan going. What's better than a ton of snuggly blankets and clean sheets? Nothing! Seriously.

- Use white noise to quiet the mind. There are so many apps that play white noise or soothing sounds to put you into your beauty sleep sooner. We love falling asleep to the tranquil sounds of the ocean or rain.

- Oil up! Essential oils are also great to use before bed. We keep a small rollerball bottle with lavender essential oil in it on the bedside table, and we apply it to our pulse points (neck, wrists, and sometimes behind the knees) when we get into bed. It helps us feel relaxed. You can also add a few drops of lavender essential oil to a diffuser so your bedroom feels like a five-star spa. Other essential oils that are good for sleep are vetiver, Roman chamomile, sandalwood, and cedarwood.

- Mini meditation. Yup, in bed! Spend a minute taking some deep breaths. Feel your legs, your arms, and your entire waistline settle into the sheets. With each breath, feel your body sink in. Breathe in slowly through your nose, hold it for a few seconds, then exhale just as slowly through your mouth. This will calm your heart rate and quiet the mind, and it's super relaxing.

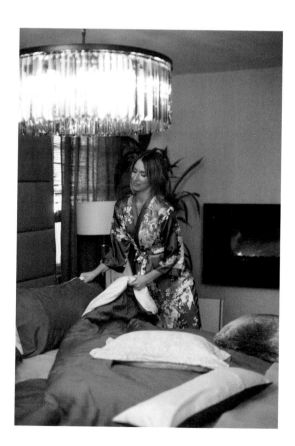

- Close your beautiful eyes and get cozy to let your mind rest. We love to use a silk sleep mask, which blocks out any extra light. Time to let your big dreams take over.

- There's always the option to un-*wine*-d too. Just a little nightcap!

YOU NEVER KNOW WHO
YOU'RE INSPIRING

We always say, "You never know who needs a little inspiration." You could be changing someone's life with just a small gesture. Think about this in everything you do!

Here are some of our favorite ways to spread love and inspiration:

- Check in with the community @ToneItUp #TIUteam. Share a sweaty selfie or meal-prep pic.

- Connect with a new babe in the community on Instagram #TIUteam or in the Studio Tone It Up app, or invite a new girlfriend to join the community.

- Invite a friend on a workout date. That's how we met, and it changed our lives forever!

- Share a healthy recipe with a girlfriend. If she doesn't normally cook, whip it up together.

- Share an inspirational quote or mantra on Instagram.

- Compliment the women around you, whether it's a friend, a coworker, or even your barista. You'll make her day! Tell someone she's lookin' gorgeous or that you've noticed how much she's been kicking booty on a project. That small amount of recognition can make a world of difference in her day.

- Post a picture on your Instagram story of someone who inspires you. You never know who needs it too!

- Volunteer. Gather a group of girlfriends and volunteer together at a local food bank, homeless shelter, children's hospital, or nursing home. You can also look up local organizations that put together charity events. Recently, I went to a yoga class where everyone brought toys for the children's hospital and local charities that support kids in need. You can also look up a local Red Cross chapter to donate blood. This is something Karena does every couple of months.

- Volunteering with friends and family is a great way to bond and give back, and there are so many opportunities to give your time and talents. We love this quote: "Kindness is magic. Sprinkle a little everywhere."

- Be a mentor. Volunteer to mentor young women, whether it's through a fitness program like Girls on the Run or through academic tutoring or mentorship.

- Be an engaged listener. Sometimes all it takes is you listening to someone to give them confidence and inspiration.

- Above all, be enthusiastic and exude love in everything you do. Your positivity will always be super inspiring and give others a boost when they need it.

inspire

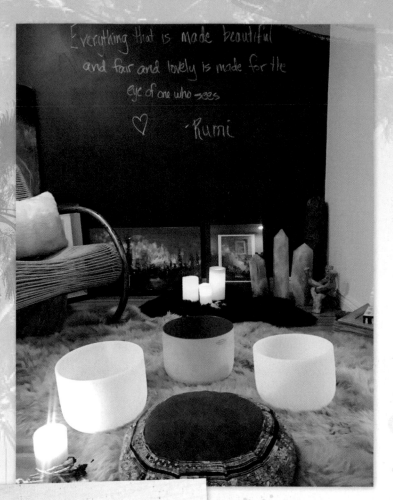

Everything that is made beautiful
and fair and lovely is made for the
eye of one who sees

♡   -Rumi

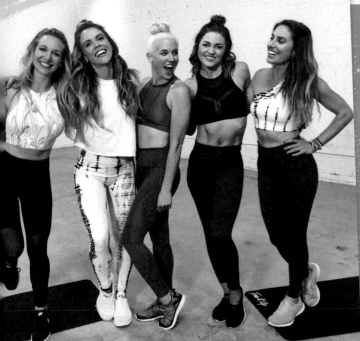

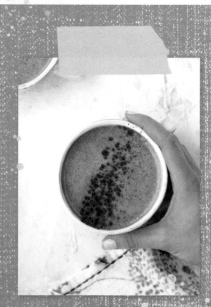

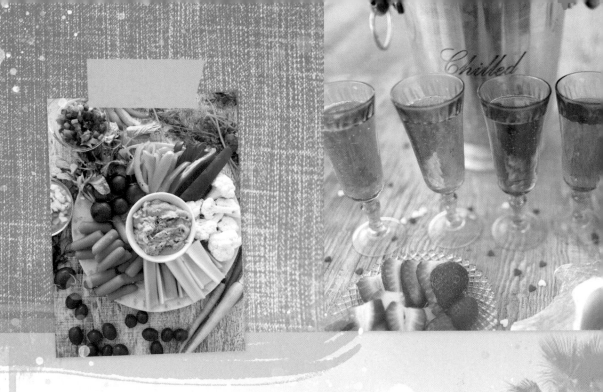

Chilled

Vision Board to Inspire

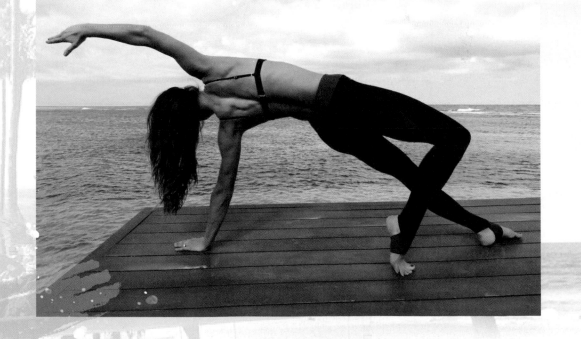

REFLECT
to Inspire

Today, I felt most inspired when I

_____

This reminds me of a time in my past when I felt really inspired.
It was when

_____

A person I find very inspiring is

_____

I'm inspired to try

_____

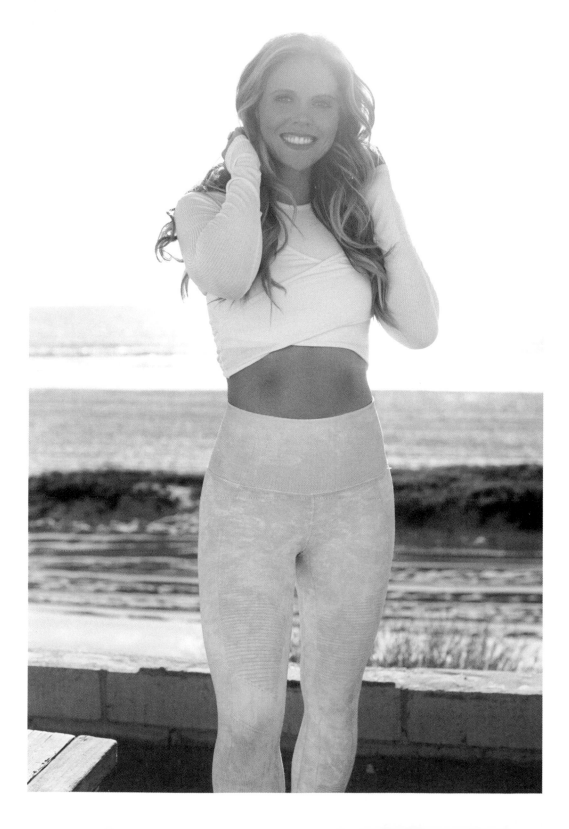

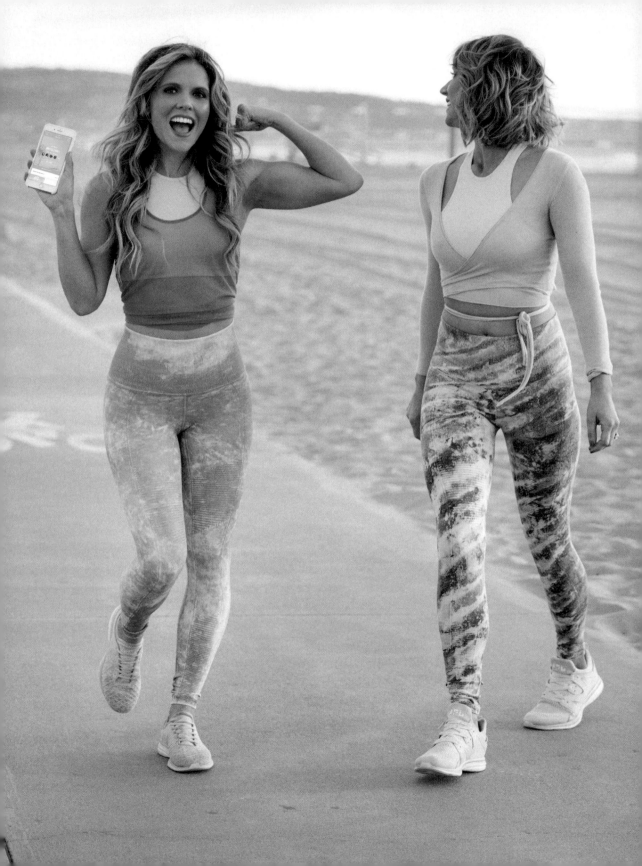

4

Energize

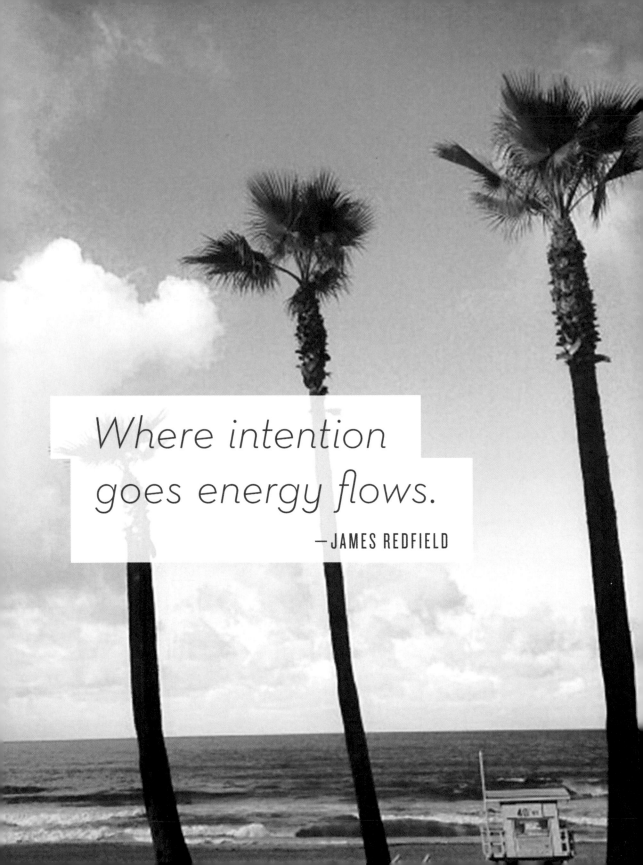

Where intention goes energy flows.

—JAMES REDFIELD

GIRL TALK
to Energize

KATRINA   Where do you draw the energy from that you need to get going and tackle your day? To us, energy is more than feeling awake—it starts with the mind and then the physical body. Having energy is feeling spirited, animated, and empowered, all of which are so important to women. Energy gives us drive and stamina in our workouts, it helps us hustle and be creative in our careers, and it allows us to give more to our loved ones. We draw energy from within ourselves, from family, friends, and community, and from caring for our bodies and treating ourselves with love.

Recently, when we were on our Tone It Up Tour, we were exhausted after thirty days of traveling and visiting fifteen cities. Aside from the thirty-six flights we took, including countless layovers and the packing and unpacking at each hotel, we were exercising our hearts out on stage and spending hours meeting tens of thousands of our girls from the community. We were so sore (like tender to the touch!) and physically spent. Even though we were tired, we were happy and fulfilled. We drew energy from the excitement and each other.

The final stop was Chicago. This was our biggest event and was at Soldier Field stadium. We got dressed, hyped ourselves up with some music, had some shots of espresso, then coconut water, then ginger and cayenne, then tequila (JK), and just starting dancing out all of our nerves. Karena does this hysterical thing where she'll start rehearsing and going through exercises in her head, and she turns it into some kind of interpretive dance. I usually get so nervous. I'm always shaking and deep breathing. It's a funny combo to witness.

As we walked out for this final stop, we didn't even need to speak. We just linked arms and made our way onto the stage. Energy spoke louder than any words we could have said to each other.

As we walked out on stage, we saw the smiling faces and beautiful, excited energy from all our girls on the field. Right there, in that moment, we had all the energy we needed, and then some.

What Energizes Me

Energy? I need coffee and Kat.

Karena

What Energizes Me

Ha-ha, *same, same, Karena!* We energize each other.

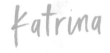
Katrina

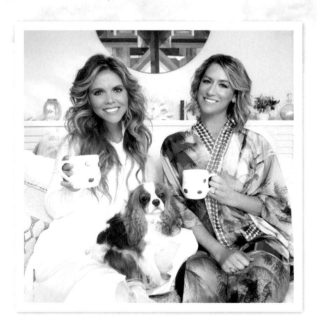

SPIRITUAL GUIDE
to Energize

Awaken Your Senses

KARENA Every morning is a new chance to start fresh, to reenergize, refocus, and reset. You don't need to wait for a new year or a new month or even a Monday! Each day you wake up and commit to yourself, you're reigniting your passions and your soul.

When we sit back and think about what makes us feel the most energized for the day, our morning always starts with awakening all five senses. You can do simple things for each sense that will help you carry that positive energy throughout your day.

Sight. See yourself and recognize how unique and amazing you are! Take a look in a mirror and say what you think, such as "I love my booty because I've worked really hard in my workouts" or "I love my freckles because they make me unique" or "I love that my arms give me the strength to pick up my kids every day." Then say three things you love about your mind and soul, such as "I love that I'm a caring and compassionate friend" or "I love that I'm striving to learn new things every day" or "I love that I'm a loving parent" or "I love that I'm taking this time to care for myself." It may seem a little unnatural to say these things aloud at first, but you deserve to hear them and you deserve to see yourself as the beautiful, brilliant, strong woman you are.

Sound. Living near the beach, we love to go for a walk in the morning and listen to the sound of the ocean. It's so restorative. No matter where you are, you can tap into the calming sounds of nature. Take a few moments to stroll around outdoors and bring awareness to your surroundings—listen to the birds, the leaves falling, a breeze . . . or maybe just the silence. When you're at home, play ambient relaxing music or Tibetan yoga music in the background to soothe you. Another incredibly refreshing thing to do is to have a "sound bath" session. A sound bath is based on an ancient tradition of refreshing and calming yourself with repetitive sounds at a certain frequency, like those from a gong or Tibetan singing bowls. If you can't find a sound bath session near you—they're usually held at meditation or yoga centers—then try YouTube or an app for guided videos.

Smell. I love to start each day by lighting candles and incense while I meditate. We talked about the benefits of incense and aromatherapy in "Refresh" (page 4). Some of my other favorite refreshing scents are vanilla (sweet and delicious, like sugar cookies!), lavender (which soothes stress), peppermint (which wakes you up and makes you feel rejuvenated), Roman chamomile (a great pick-me-up to boost your mood), grapefruit (the tangy scent gets you out the door and on the move), and eucalyptus (which helps you feel refreshed if you're having a hard time getting going in the morning).

Taste. Start each day with foods that detoxify your body and make you feel lean, light, and energized. Try Kat's Matcha Latte Bowl (page 162), or pick from some of our favorites in "Detoxifying Foods and Sips" (page 18).

Touch. An easy way to start off the day refreshed and detoxed is to spend a few minutes giving yourself a DIY at-home reflexology session. Your hands and feet are full of super-sensitive nerves, and reflexology works by applying pressure to specific areas that correspond to different conditions that may be bothering you. Reflexology can also help detoxify the body and stimulate the digestive system. One study showed that female undergraduate students who practiced reflexology three times a week felt less stressed, and it improved their energy levels.

Reflexology is easy to do at home by using a standardized map of the feet and/or hands, such as the one on page 146, which shows the areas of the feet that correspond to all the organs, glands, and other parts of the body.

Try this simple ten-minute routine from Laura Norman, a board-certified reflexologist and author of the bestselling book *Feet First: A Guide to Foot Reflexology*. This routine is perfect to do before your workout or right after you get out of the shower:

1. Relax your feet with simple relaxation techniques: pressing, squeezing, *lightly* slapping, gently kneading—whatever feels good.

2. On the bottom of each foot, "walk" your thumb up from the base of the heel to each toe using tiny movements (imagine your thumb as a caterpillar inching up your foot).

3. If your feet are sore, spend more time on relaxation techniques and then gently press the following points on the bottom of each foot with your thumb or index finger for five to ten seconds each (see the chart):

REFLEXOLOGY CHART

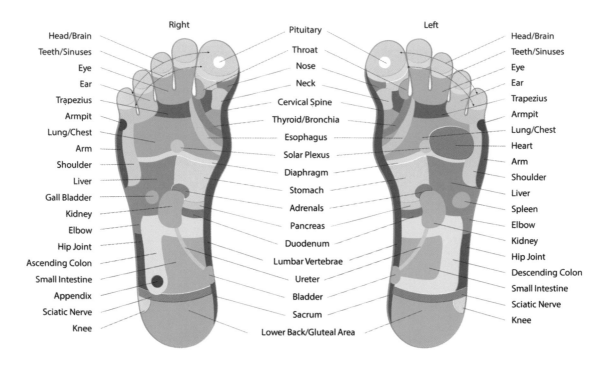

Right		Left
Head/Brain	Pituitary	Head/Brain
Teeth/Sinuses	Throat	Teeth/Sinuses
Eye	Nose	Eye
Ear	Neck	Ear
Trapezius	Cervical Spine	Trapezius
Armpit	Thyroid/Bronchia	Armpit
Lung/Chest	Esophagus	Lung/Chest
Arm	Solar Plexus	Heart
Shoulder	Diaphragm	Arm
Liver	Stomach	Shoulder
Gall Bladder	Adrenals	Liver
Kidney	Pancreas	Spleen
Elbow	Duodenum	Elbow
Hip Joint	Lumbar Vertebrae	Kidney
Ascending Colon	Ureter	Hip Joint
Small Intestine	Bladder	Descending Colon
Appendix	Sacrum	Small Intestine
Sciatic Nerve	Lower Back/Gluteal Area	Sciatic Nerve
Knee		Knee

Pituitary gland—stimulates production of endorphins and balances hormone secretions of many other glands

Shoulder and arm—enhances flexibility and performance

Lung/chest—opens the airways for deeper breathing

Solar plexus—reduces stress and relaxes breathing

Adrenals—produce cortisone/cortisol to reduce inflammation and adrenaline to boost energy

Cervical spine—balances the nervous system (walk from the heel to the base of the big toenail)

Sciatic nerve—improves circulation to the lower back and legs

4. Repeat the relaxation techniques. Finish with another thumb press on the solar plexus points on both feet.

5. End with "breeze strokes"—lightly run your fingertips down the tops, bottoms, and sides of each foot in a feathery motion, barely touching the skin. These are so soothing.

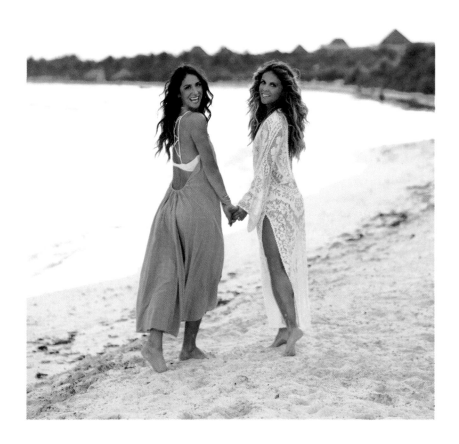

WORKOUT GUIDE
to Energize

Exercise gives you a huge energy boost. Between the endorphins, your heart rate rising, the increase in your stamina, and just the feeling of moving your body, working out is one of the best ways to actually gain energy for the rest of your day. Plus, you'll have a beautiful rosy glow.

We love HIIT in particular for a quick rush of energy!

Energize with High-Intensity Interval Training

Complete *three circuits* of the following moves, doing as many reps as you can in 30 seconds for each one, and take *a 30-second break between* the sets:

1 *Jump Tuck*

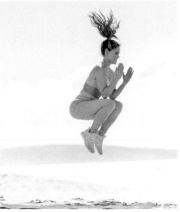

2 *Squat and Leg Abduction*

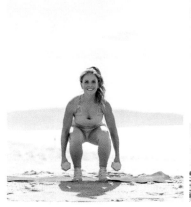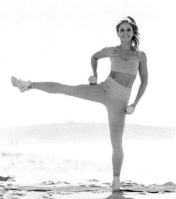

3 *Jumping Jacks*

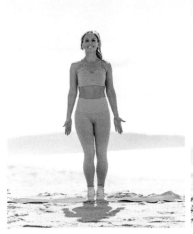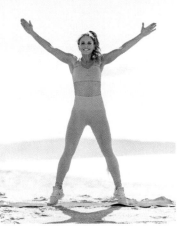

energize

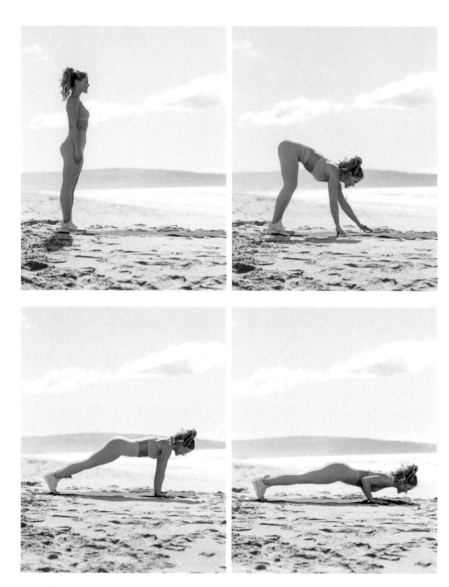

 Bikini Walk Out and Push-Up

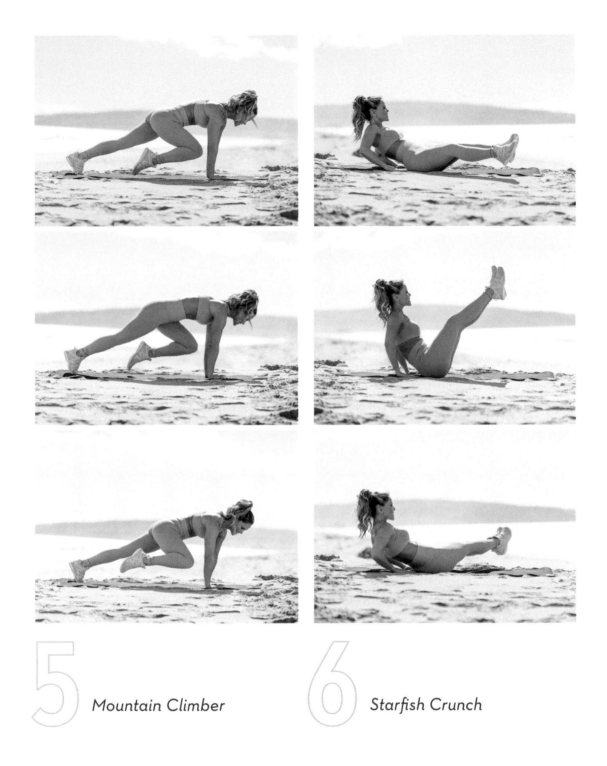

5 Mountain Climber

6 Starfish Crunch

energize

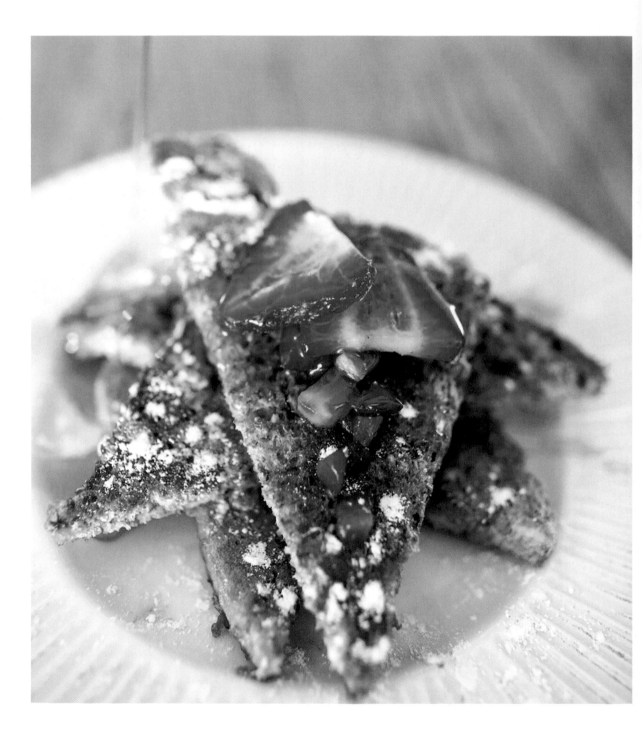

RECIPE GUIDE
to Energize

There's no doubt that eating gives you energy, but some foods can actually leave you in a slump. The secret to eating foods that will energize you is making sure the foods are clean and easy for your body to digest. If a meal is too dense and unhealthy, you'll notice yourself feeling run-down, because your digestive system needs to step in and work in overdrive. With the following recipes you'll feel satisfied, light, refreshed, and ready to kick some major booty!

FRENCHY TOAST

Serves 1

1 teaspoon coconut oil, or coconut oil spray

¼ cup egg whites

1 tablespoon vanilla Tone It Up Protein

½ teaspoon ground cinnamon

2 slices Ezekiel bread

Strawberries, honey, or maple syrup (optional)

Melt the coconut oil in a large pan, or coat the pan with coconut oil spray. Heat the pan on a medium setting.

In a bowl, whisk together the egg whites, Tone It Up Protein, and cinnamon.

Dip both sides of each piece of bread in the mixture, then transfer the soaked bread to the hot pan.

Cook each side of the bread for 2 minutes, or until they are golden brown.

Serve the Frenchy Toast plain or topped with strawberries, honey, or maple syrup.

SIMPLE SUPERFOOD BARS

Makes 9

1/2 cup unsweetened almond butter

1 tablespoon coconut oil, melted

2 tablespoons honey

1/4 cup vanilla Tone It Up Protein

1/2 cup unsweetened coconut flakes

1/2 cup chopped almonds

1/4 cup goji berries (or other superfood of choice)

1/4 cup cacao nibs

Coconut oil spray

Stir the almond butter and coconut oil together in a medium or large bowl. Add the honey, Tone It Up Protein, coconut flakes, chopped almonds, goji berries, and cacao nibs, and stir until everything is well combined.

Coat a 9 × 13-inch baking dish with coconut oil spray, then press the mixture into the dish.

Refrigerate the bars until you are ready to eat them. At that time, cut them into 9 equal portions.

VANILLA LATTE SMOOTHIE

Serves 1

1/2 cup unsweetened almond milk ice cubes

3/4 cup unsweetened almond milk

1 shot espresso

1 scoop vanilla Tone It Up Protein

1/2 cup frozen banana slices (optional, for a creamier consistency)

In a high-speed blender, combine all the ingredients until the mixture is smooth. Enjoy!

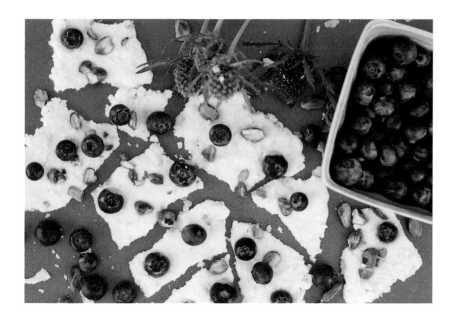

BLUEBERRY COCONUT BARK

Serves 8

1 1/2 cups unsweetened coconut flakes

1 tablespoon coconut oil

1/4 cup fresh blueberries

3 tablespoons chopped pistachios

Blend the coconut flakes and coconut oil in a food processor until the mixture is smooth. This could take 3 to 7 minutes.

On a cookie sheet lined with parchment paper or foil, spread the coconut mixture in a thin circular layer. It should take up about half a standard-size cookie sheet.

Gently press the blueberries and pistachios into the coconut mixture.

Freeze the mixture for 3 to 4 hours, then break it into 8 roughly equal-size pieces before serving.

energize

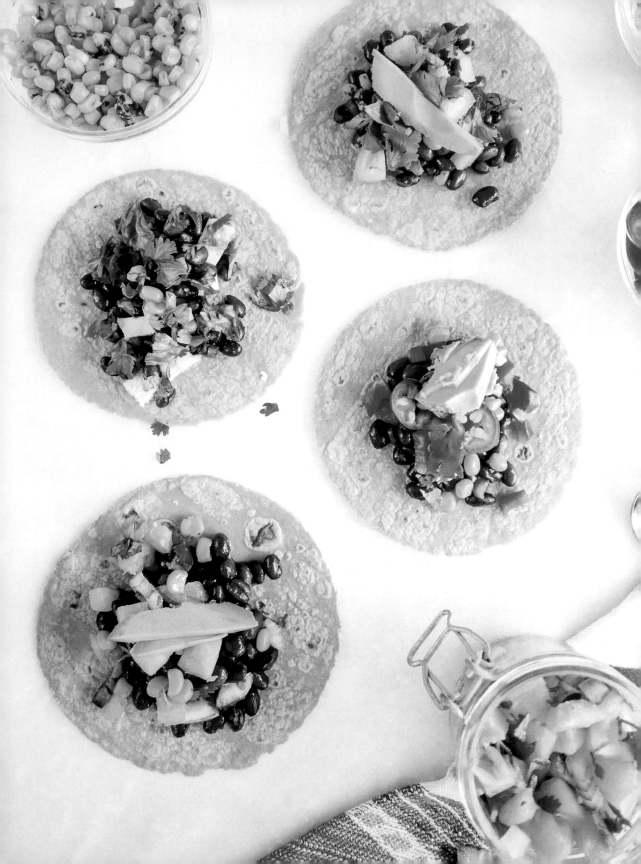

Taco Tuesday Inspo!

TACO 'BOUT IT

Serves 2

½ cup canned pinto or black beans, drained and rinsed

1 teaspoon coconut oil

4 corn tortillas

½ cup shredded romaine lettuce

½ cup diced red onion

½ avocado, peeled, pitted, and diced

¼ cup corn

½ jalapeño, thinly sliced

½ cup Pineapple Salsa (page 69)

1 small bunch cilantro, chopped

Hot sauce of your choice, to taste (optional)

In a pan, sauté the beans in the coconut oil until they are warm.

Place the tortillas on a plate, then top them with the beans, lettuce, onion, avocado, corn, jalapeño, salsa, cilantro, and hot sauce, if using.

CILANTRO LIME GUACAMOLE

Serves 4

2 avocados, peeled and pitted

¼ cup diced red onion

¼ cup chopped

fresh cilantro

Juice of 1 lime

Pinch of salt

In a small or medium bowl, combine all the ingredients, mashing everything with a fork until the guacamole is a desired consistency. Serve the guacamole with sliced cucumbers and carrots or any other veggies you like.

energize

ARROZ CON POLLO

Serves 4

1 tablespoon coconut oil

4 6-ounce chicken breasts

¼ teaspoon salt

1 yellow onion, diced

4 cloves garlic, chopped

1 red bell pepper, chopped

¼ teaspoon ground paprika

½ cup tomato sauce

¾ cups brown rice or quinoa

1 ½ cups vegetable broth

½ cup frozen peas

In a large pot or pan set over medium heat, melt the coconut oil. Add the chicken and sprinkle each breast with salt. Cook the chicken breasts on both sides for 6 to 8 minutes, then transfer them to a plate.

To the same pot or pan, add the onion, garlic, bell pepper, paprika, and tomato sauce, and sauté the mixture for about 4 minutes.

Add the rice or quinoa and the broth, and bring everything to a boil, then reduce the heat. Simmer the mixture, covered, for 25 minutes.

Return the chicken breasts to the pot or pan. Simmer, covered, for an additional 15 minutes.

Stir the peas into the pot, and simmer, covered, for another 5 minutes, then serve.

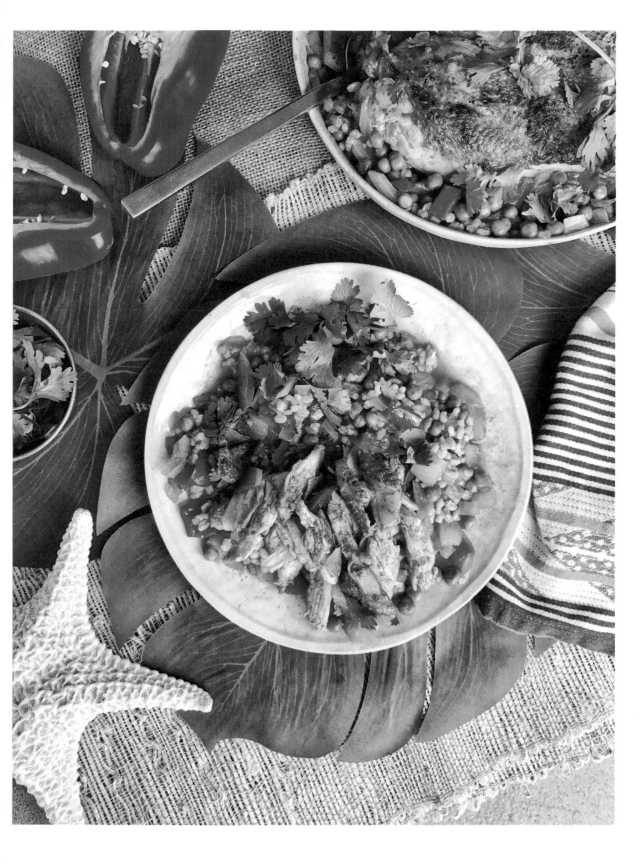

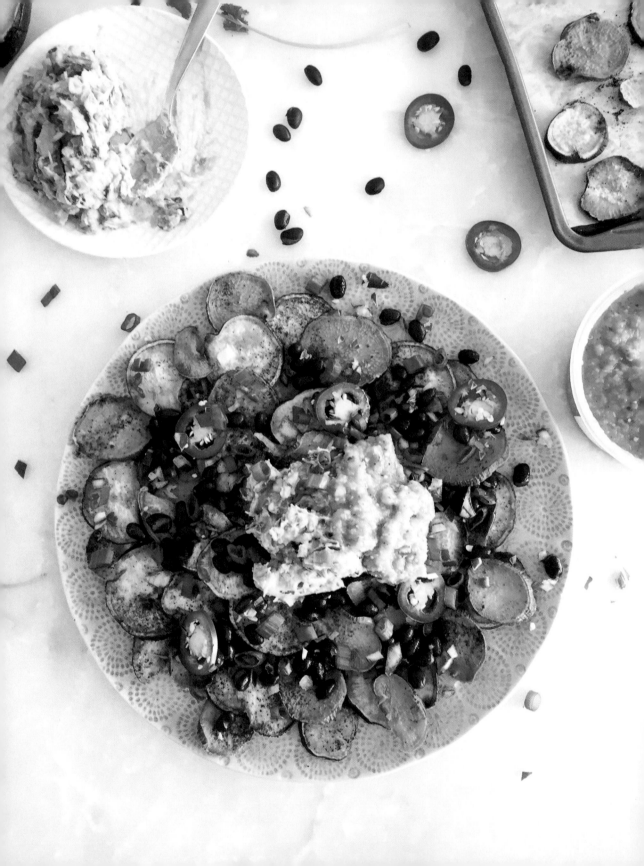

NACHO AVERAGE NACHOS

Serves 6

2 sweet potatoes, peeled and thinly sliced

4 teaspoons olive oil

2 teaspoons chili powder

2 pinches salt

1 15-ounce can black beans, drained and rinsed

½ cup green salsa

¼ cup chopped fresh cilantro

3 tablespoons chopped chives or green onion

2 tablespoons finely diced red onion

1 jalapeño, thinly sliced

FOR THE HOT 'N' SPICY GUACAMOLE

2 avocados, peeled and pitted

½ jalapeño, finely diced

3 tablespoons chopped fresh cilantro

Juice of ½ lemon

Pinch of salt

Preheat the oven to 400°F.

Spread the sweet potato slices on two baking sheets covered with parchment paper. Drizzle the potatoes with the olive oil, and sprinkle them with the chili powder and salt. Toss to coat all the slices. Roast the potatoes for 15 minutes, or until they reach a desired crispness.

While the potatoes are roasting, prepare the guacamole. In a bowl, mash together all the guacamole ingredients well, then set it aside.

Transfer the sweet potato chips to a large platter. Top them with the black beans, green salsa, cilantro, chives or green onion, red onion, jalapeño, and ½ cup of the guacamole. (You can use the extra guac for dipping with veggies.)

Extra servings can be stored in the fridge for up to four days.

energize

SPICY GRAPEFRUIT MARGARITAS

Serves 2

Juice of 1 large grapefruit

2 ounces tequila

1 ounce triple sec or Cointreau

1 jalapeño, sliced

1 teaspoon honey

Ice

Margarita salt and/or low-sodium chili lime seasoning

In a jar or mixed-drink shaker, shake up the grapefruit juice, tequila, triple sec or Cointreau, sliced jalapeño, and honey with some ice for 10 to 15 seconds.

Rim 2 glasses with margarita salt and/or low-sodium chili lime seasoning.

Pour the cocktail over ice. ¡Salud!

KAT'S MATCHA LATTE BOWL

Serves 1

1 cup unsweetened almond milk

1 scoop vanilla Tone It Up Protein

1/2 cup chopped frozen pineapple

1/2 frozen banana, sliced

1 teaspoon matcha

2 tablespoons almond yogurt

Toppings (optional):
1 tablespoon coconut flakes, cacao nibs, or goji berries, or 1 sliced kiwi fruit

In a high-speed blender, puree the almond milk, Tone It Up Protein, pineapple, and banana until the mixture is smooth. Pour it into a bowl.

In a separate bowl, stir together the matcha and almond yogurt until they are well combined. Drizzle this mixture over your smoothie bowl.

Sprinkle on any of the optional toppings, if you like.

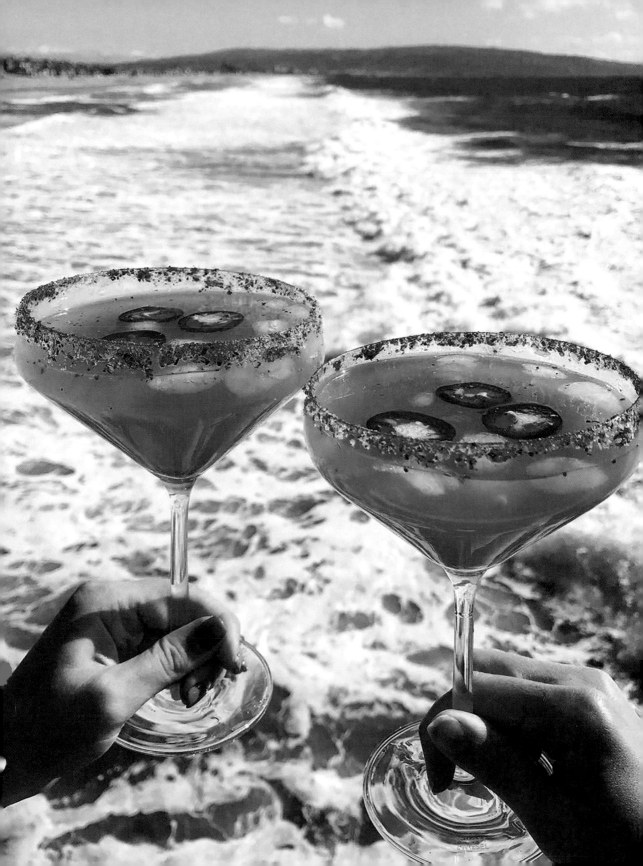

EAT YOUR HEART OUT!

Looking for the most nutritious, energizing foods? Choose whole, unprocessed lean, clean, 'n' green options. Colorful fruits and vegetables will deliver restorative vitamins and minerals. You also want to opt for complex carbohydrates and lean proteins that will sustain you during your workouts and all day long. Here are our top choices:

- Guac is extra . . . but so am I. Add that *avocado*. High-quality, heart-healthy monounsaturated fat in avocados helps slow digestion, so you don't get any energy spikes or crashes.

- Egg-cellent! Containing protein and healthy fats, *eggs* deliver choline, part of the B-complex vitamins that support your energy level and boost your metabolism.

- Be a green goddess: dark, leafy *greens* like kale are a powerhouse of vitamins and minerals, like folate, vitamin C, and beta-carotene, which fight fatigue and replenish the body in times of stress.

- Are you a chocolate lover? Pure unsweetened *cacao* is full of energizing antioxidants and can improve your circulation and lower your blood pressure. We love smoothie bowls made with chocolate Tone It Up Protein and sprinkled with cacao nibs.

- O-mega babe! *Salmon* is packed with heart-healthy omega-3 fatty acids as well as high levels of vitamin B_{12} to boost your energy level.

- Pronounced "keen-wah," *quinoa* is actually a seed, but it cooks and tastes just like a grain. We love quinoa because it gives you a nice balance of carbohydrate and protein. It also contains nearly twice as much fiber as most grains.

- Go nuts. *Almonds* deliver fiber, magnesium, and B vitamins, which keep your energy level up through the afternoon. Grab a handful around 4 p.m.

- Or go bananas. Containing fiber, *bananas* will keep your energy level steady without any crashes. Plus, they're loaded with potassium to help you recover post-workout. We slice and freeze them every Sunday to use in smoothies all week.

- *Oats* are one of our favorite breakfasts. They are filled with fiber that aids digestion and reduces energy spikes and crashes. We like to make a batch of overnight oats on Sunday and store them in mason jars to grab 'n' go in the morning.

- Love you so matcha. *Matcha* is a top-quality green tea, but the leaves have been ground into a fine, bright green powder, which gives it a much higher concentration of caffeine and antioxidants since you're ingesting the whole leaf, not just steeping it. We love matcha stirred into smoothies, almond milk, and even baked treats like muffins.

energize

GIRLFRIEND GUIDE
to Energize

KATRINA   Close your eyes and think about the friends in your life who energize you. Who energetically supports you? Who lifts you up and makes you want to get out and seize the day? What qualities do they have? What about them do you want to emulate so you can return that incredible power back to them?

I can't count the times when I've been so exhausted and my friends come in to save the day and boost me. When I feel like curling up in a ball for the weekend after a long week of work, they bring out the best in me and urge me to get out and enjoy all that life has to offer! No one ever regrets making memories—so I put together some of the top girlfriend dates that will energize you any day of the week. Just figure out when you're available, and plan anything from this list:

Sunday Fun Day! We all know a Sunday full of laundry, meal prep, and cleaning is productive, but the truth is, I don't remember any of them from last summer. I only remember the bike rides to brunch, the fun hikes that led to an early dinner at our favorite spot, the tailgating, the double sessions of yoga sculpt and healthy meal prep together with friends, the family trip to the beach, the happy hour and karaoke combo . . . Seriously, sometimes you just need an energetic Sunday Fun Day to fuel your week. Try to stay on top of your home to-do list so you can enjoy your Sunday . . . and make memories for the week.

> *"Off to make memories for our group chat this week . . ."*

Move It Monday! Mondays can be a bit crazy, so planning short bursts of energy throughout the day is key. Ask your coworkers or girlfriends to meet up for a quick coffee chat at a coffee shop. Lunchtime? Get outside for a short fifteen-minute walk to get moving. Afternoon slump? Energize yourself with some stairs—hit the stairs in your office, outside, or in your house. Getting the blood flowing throughout your entire body will awaken your brain to crush the last hours of your Monday. Home late? Join a Studio Tone It Up class and work it out with the community!

> *"I love it when the coffee kicks in and I realize what an adorable badass I'm going to be."*

Taco Tuesday! Sometimes I can't wait for the weekend and it's only Tuesday. Mondays and Tuesdays can be long—twenty hours of work and hustle—so a little break during the week is just what the girlfriend ordered. Head out for an hour or two and just connect and taco 'bout it. (Yup, I had to . . .)

> *"Don't tell me you're thinking of me. . . .*
> *Show up outside in a taco truck."*

Workout Wednesday! In the "Motivate" chapter, we talked about accountability and meeting up for classes. Hump day is the perfect day to sign up for a high-energy class. Think heart pumping, fun, and memorable. Meet up for a dance class, hip-hop, cycling, trapeze (Karena and I did this and it was so much fun!!), an aerial silk class (we've been wanting to try this), Pound (where you work out with drumsticks and feel like a total rocker!), boot camp, boxing, circuit training (we've been seeing

energize

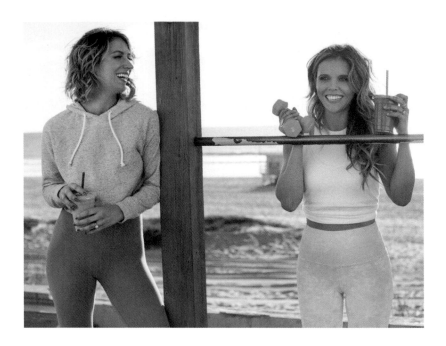

so many where they dim the lights and blast music), Zumba, pole (where you dance on a pole—whether it's your thing or not, it's hysterical and so much fun to do with girlfriends; Neicee from TIU HQ does it every week!), yoga on paddleboards, or go on a run with new scenery, like at a local stadium—sometimes the best things in life are free!

> *"I really regret that workout . . .*
> *said no one ever."*

Teach Me Thursday! We love learning new things. Karena and I have taken fun classes, like etiquette (we failed miserably, LOL), art, and golf. You can also look for pottery (I used to go every Thursday), sewing (my mom used to teach sewing—she's a seamstress and it was so much fun), musical instruments, singing, cooking, jewelry making, private dance classes, flower arranging, macramé, gardening (I need to do this ASAP), cooking, surfing, paddleboarding, synchronized swimming (ha-ha—yup, we thought of it), makeup application, perfume making (Karena and I just did this in Venice Beach, and it was one of the coolest things!), acting or other performance arts, tennis, volleyball (or any other sport), woodshop (my friend Katie just built her own bed—not even kidding—and it's beautiful), paint and vino night, or you can make it into a Thirsty Thursday and learn about wine!

"Every day should be a new adventure: say yes."

Friday—A League of Their Own! This is a fun one that a lot of our girls at TIU HQ do. Join an athletic team, such as a run club, kickball league, or volleyball team. You can also turn it into a volunteer team and join a Big Sisters program, clean the beach or parks, paint schools, or volunteer at your local YMCA.

"Okay, let's make like a bread truck
and haul buns, ladies!"
—FROM *A LEAGUE OF THEIR OWN*

Salsa Saturday! There are so many fun places where you can go dancing with your girls. Hit the town for a salsa night or line dancing. It's also a fun thing to do on a double-date.

"Trust me, you can dance.
xo, Margarita."

energize

BEAUTY TIPS
to Energize

KARENA   There are so many ways you can boost your mood and energy just by adding something to your beauty routine, or by wearing something different. Do you ever notice you have more energy during your workout if you feel confident? Do you notice yourself standing taller and walking with more pep in your step at work when your hair is blown out and you're wearing your favorite outfit? For me, just a pop of fuchsia on my lips will make me come alive any day.

Here are a few ways to energize your look immediately:

- Enjoy a cooling under-eye mask.

- Put eucalyptus or citrus oil on your wrists.

- Rub in a tropical lotion . . . everywhere
  (the smell brings me back to Hawaii).

- Use an energetic nail and lip color.

- A high pony be poppin'!

- Or do half pony and half Bamm-Bamm hair!

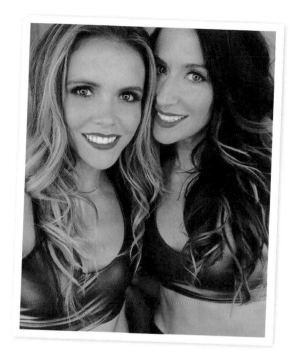

- Apply a li'l brow, li'l mascara, li'l bronzer and blush . . . and highlighter.

- Try cat eyes: wing it—it's what all angels do.

- Tight-line your lower lash line with a light tan to offset any redness, then add highlighter in between your eyes.

- Go for a coral top. Wearing orange tones will actually energize you, and everyone around you.

energize

CONNECT WITH THE TONE IT UP COMMUNITY
to Energize

The Tone It Up community is made up of so many busy women—boss babes, mamas, students—who balance their careers and families, and dedicate time to their health with positivity and grace. We asked some of these incredible women to share their advice on how to stay energized in the morning and all day long.

Stories from Community Members

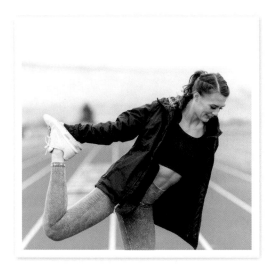

Elise

Elise @eliselefit

"My first tip would be to hydrate! Making sure I have enough water is a must. I feel better and my skin looks brighter all day long. Eat every two to three hours! If I go too long without food, I get "hangry"! I make sure I am always packing snacks for those long days. And always try to get a morning workout in. I have found I am a happier and nicer person all day long if I got in a good sweat in the morning. I have more patience for myself and those around me."

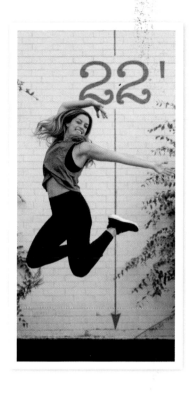

Morgan

Morgan @bunundone

"Since I work at a desk, screen time really takes a toll on my eyes, and sitting takes a toll on my body. During the day, I make sure to take some walking breaks to keep my body and blood flow moving, whether it's to chat face-to-face with a coworker or fill up on my water, and it helps a ton with my energy level. Tea has been a huge factor for me as well! After lunch, I love sipping on green tea to help me digest as well as provide a slight energy boost."

Natasha

Natasha @making_fit_count

"Make sure you're fueling your body throughout the day. Stay hydrated, get adequate amounts of your macronutrients, carbs, healthy fats, and proteins, and always do your best to take a step back and breathe when you're feeling overwhelmed. I used to be so drained midday, but ever since I started doing these few things, I've noticed my energy lasts longer, and I rarely feel tired during the day anymore."

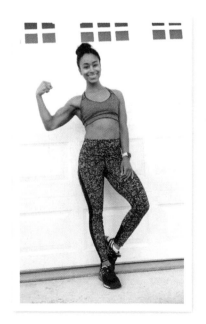

energize

Community Member Moms

TIU moms share their best tips for staying energized while caring for their little ones!

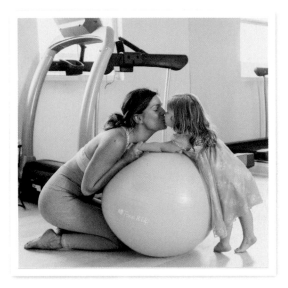

Ashley

Ashley @ashbrookedaily

"Making time for myself first thing in the morning, setting my intentions for the day, and sweating for my strength and soul make me better in all the hats I wear: mom, wife, leader, and friend. My best tips for other moms who are looking to make time for themselves in the morning are to share your 'why' with your partner or spouse and get them on your team! My husband is my biggest cheerleader; he will ask me if I got my daily moves in! And be flexible! Every week may look slightly different. On Sundays, take some time to look at the upcoming week and identify any potential challenges or disruptions to your normal routine. Is there something you can shift around? Is there a day that maybe you have to give up your extra hour of TV for the extra hour of sleep so you can get up earlier? Assess your week and go in with a plan! And finally, *stay positive*! Being negative is *exhausting*. No matter how busy you are, no matter how crazy your toddler is being, *you* are here, *you* are healthy, and *you* are showing up for yourself every single day, and that's pretty amazing. Seek out the positivity in every situation and it will help you stay energized all day long!"

Terra

Terra @terratonesitup

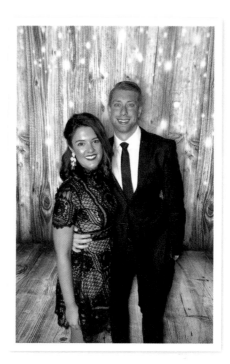

"Some of my best advice is to wake up thirty minutes before your family. This gives you time for yourself before the rest of the world starts moving. I love how quiet this time is, and how it sets the tone for the day. By prepping lunches and coffee and working out before everyone else is awake, I'm able to be present once the rest of the family is up. This makes for a much smoother transition into the school and work day.

"And don't forget to laugh daily and have fun! Have a family dance party, invite your girlfriends over for game night, watch your favorite rom-com, plan an active date night. Smiling and laughing make every day better!"

energize

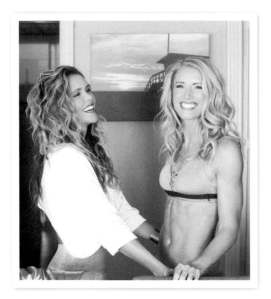

Whitney

Whitney @whitfit.tiu

"I am a stay-at-home mom to my toddler son, so I need all of the energy I can get! Chasing after him is an added workout but such a blessing. I love to start my morning routine with a cup of green tea as I set my intentions and have my spiritual time before my workout. During my workouts, I love to diffuse essential oils that keep me focused and energized! For me, this routine fuels my heart, body, and soul with the energy I need to feel balanced in all of life's chaos through the day!

"If you feel there is ever too much on your plate and you feel you need to recharge, don't be afraid to ask for help! We as mamas and boss babes often tend to view asking for help as a sign of weakness. Do you have a significant other, grandparent, sibling, or friend that would love a few extra hours with your little one? Don't be afraid to *ask*! Take this time to get a few things done off your to-do list. Whether it is meal prepping a few meals for the week, going for a long run, getting a mani, catching up with a friend, and by all means . . . time to relax! Tone It Up helped me realize that there is nothing wrong with taking time to love *yourself*. Giving myself this time each day has allowed me to exude more love and joy toward myself and my family, and to feel capable of keeping up with the hustle and bustle of mom life."

ACTION GUIDE
to Energize

Want to wake up on the right side of the bed each day? Us too! Having a great morning leads to a great day—and it all starts with your morning routine. So here it goes.

Our Favorite Tips to Get Your Booty Out of Bed and Energize You for the Day

- You snooze, you lose! Set your alarm clock across the room so you literally have to hop out of bed to turn it off. Call us crazy, but it works! It makes it so much harder to hit that SNOOZE button—and to sit in bed and cruise Instagram for twenty minutes! Yeah, we're all guilty of that from time to time. Plus, did you know that hitting SNOOZE can actually make you more tired because you fall back into your sleep cycle? Once you've gone a week or so without hitting SNOOZE, your body will adjust and you'll start your day with so much more energy. Good mornin', sunshine!

- Open up! Before you go to bed, open your curtains. Your body has an internal clock that resets itself with the morning sun. You'll stop producing the sleep hormone melatonin once you see the sun shine through. Sunshine is also a great source of vitamin D, which naturally boosts your energy level.

- Wake up and drink up! Your body is usually dehydrated in the morning, so be sure to drink a glass of water as soon as you get up. We like to keep a big water bottle on our bedside table so it's the first thing we do.

MORNING MOCHA

Serves 1

This is one of our favorite smoothies to make before an intense morning workout. Headed out the door with no breakfast? This is perfect for that too. It's a two-fer deal, with energy and coffee in one!

½ cup sliced frozen banana

2 teaspoons whole espresso beans or grounds

1 scoop chocolate Tone It Up Protein

1 cup ice cubes

1 shot espresso or ½ cup coffee

½ cup unsweetened almond milk

In a high-speed blender, blend all the ingredients, and wake up!

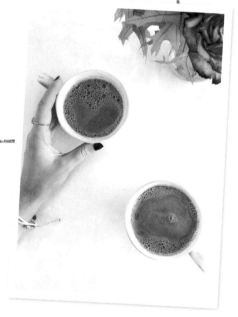

- Exercise early! We call this your booty call—wake up and work that booty! We like to get our workout done before distractions come up. No matter what comes your way during the day, your workout will make you feel balanced, centered, and energized. Also, research shows that exercising in the morning boosts your metabolism for the entire day, so you'll be burning up and glowing as you sit at your desk or hustle around town. Plus, exercise releases your brain's feel-good fuel, serotonin and dopamine, which will make you feel happier and more productive throughout the day.

   If your schedule doesn't allow for a full workout in the morning, that's okay. Just aim to get moving in some way. Walk ten minutes away from your house and ten minutes back with your morning coffee. You can even do this while you're setting your daily intentions or calling your mom or best friend to check in. Whatever works best for you, your schedule, and your body is what gives you the best results.

- There's nothing better than waking up to the smell of freshly brewed coffee. If you have a coffee machine with a timer, set it to start a few minutes before your alarm goes off so it'll be ready when you get out of bed. For an iced brew, pre-make a batch and store it in a large mason jar in the fridge. You can prep enough for up to four days. In the morning, pour yourself a glass over ice, and you're ready to go. Fun tip: if you make coffee ice cubes, they won't water down your drink!

   We also love putting coffee in our Tone It Up bottle or any other insulated reusable thermos, which will keep it cold or hot. We bring one on our java walks—plus it saves time and money. If you're not a coffee person, matcha does the trick: try Kat's Matcha Latte Bowl (page 162).

- Pump it up in the morning! Make a playlist to listen to while you get ready for the day. It's hard *not* to move when the music is so energizing. See our "Balanced and Beautiful" playlists on Spotify at Tone It Up.

- Resist the temptation to run right to the computer or phone to check all your messages. This is your time and you deserve it! If you really concentrate on yourself without distractions, you're going to be so much more energized, focused, and creative after your morning routine.

- If you're a night owl and find it hard to wake up bright and early, go easy on yourself. Everyone has a different internal clock, and some need more time to adjust. That's totally natural. Make small changes gradually. Hit the sheets ten minutes earlier and wake up ten minutes earlier. You can handle ten minutes! Once you've adjusted, add ten more minutes. Before you know it, you'll have a new morning routine and it will feel like second nature.

Evening Steps for Success

On a good evening, we'll do everything in the following list. We totally understand that after work commitments, events, and dinner dates, sometimes there is no time for it all, but here are some #eveninggoals:

- We mentioned laying out your workout clothes for the day. If you want to take this a step further, you can also rearrange your closet to make sure that your leggings, sports bras, socks, and sneakers are in the most accessible spots so you don't have to go digging for them early in the morning.

- It always helps to set aside your outfit for the day the night before too—this way you don't have to decide in a rush.

- Pack your purse and any other bags with everything you need for the day so it's ready to grab 'n' go in the morning.

KEEP THE ENERGY
FLOWING AT WORK

KATRINA Feeling an afternoon slump coming on? Get moving! I love to do spontaneous squats at my desk. If I have a meeting with someone and we're just chatting, I'll ask them to go for a quick walk with me. Sometimes we end up getting more creative ideas just from being outside! Whenever she can, Karena walks the talk—she'll take calls outside.

As soon as your body is in motion, your brain is refueled, your core wakes up, and your energy level rises. You'll feel even more focused to get back into action and continue being the total boss babe that you are!

- No blowout in the morning! To save time, at night when your hair is still damp, put it in a loose French braid. When you wake up, take it out and use sea salt spray and a little dry shampoo. If some curls in the front need to be touched up, wrap those areas around a low-heat iron to curl them away from your face. Hello, Farrah Fawcett waves!

- Break-*fast*: get all your smoothie ingredients ready the night before and keep them in a mason jar in the fridge (or if you have a NutriBullet, you can put them in the unit's container). Then all you need to do is blend them in the morning.

- Resist the temptation to look at your emails or do too much Instagram browsing in the evening. You're winding down, remember. Save your energy for tomorrow—now it's time to get into bed for a deep, refreshing sleep after your energy-fueled day.

energize

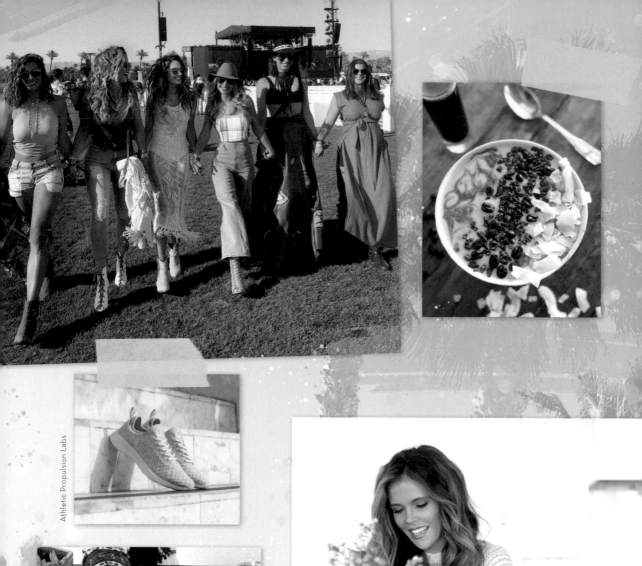

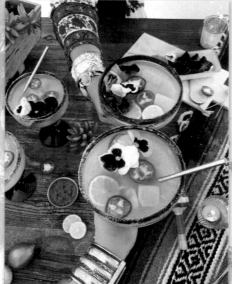

Athletic Propulsion Labs

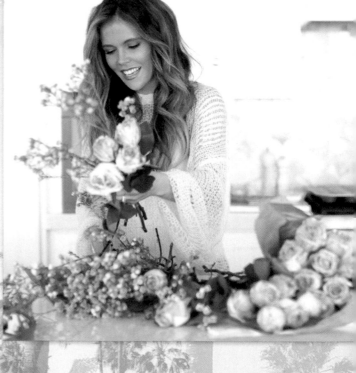

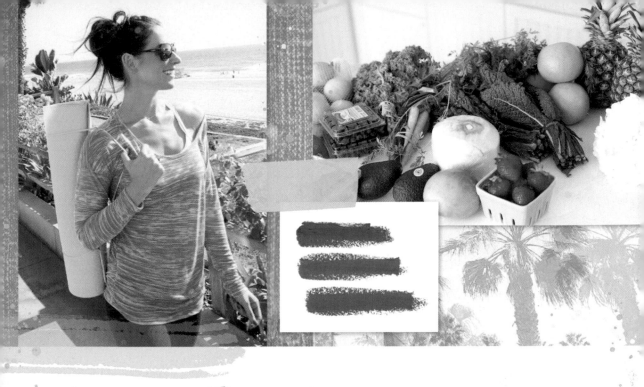

Vision Board to Energize

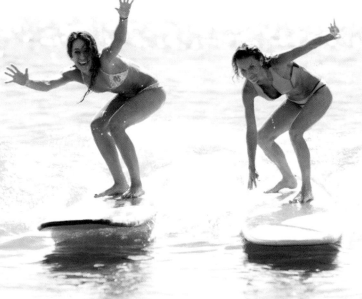

REFLECT
to Energize

The time of day I feel most energized is

_____

My favorite energizing food or drink is

_____

Someone whose energy I admire is

_____

When I have more energy I'll be able to accomplish

_____

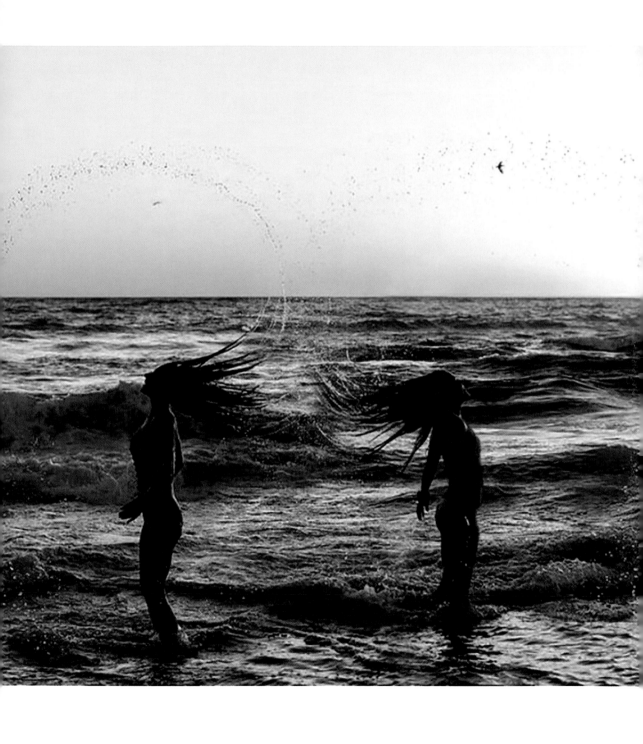

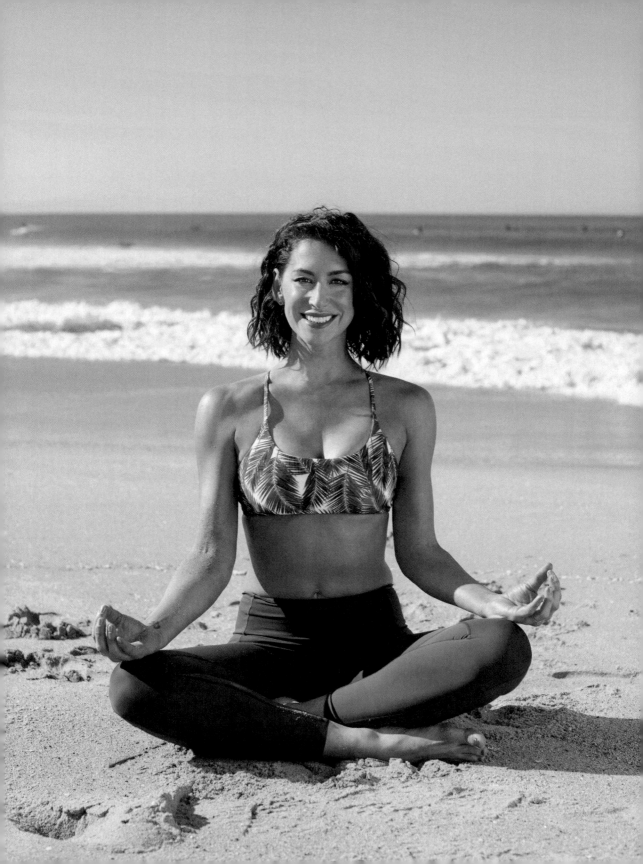

5

Relax

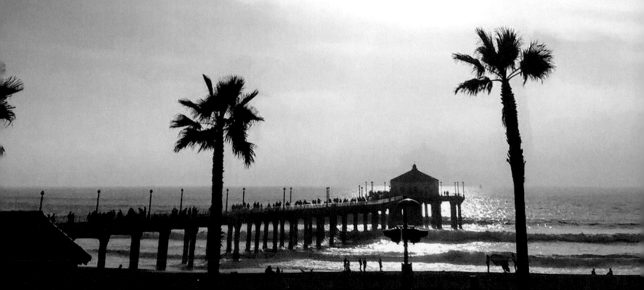

Sometimes the most important thing in a whole day is the rest we take between two deep breaths.

—ETTY HILLESUM

GIRL TALK
to Relax

Thinking back—on all the work we've done, the trips we've been on together, the places we've seen, the countries we've traveled to, and the beautiful experiences we've been so lucky to go through together— we've always made time to relax with each other. Our quality time is spent soaking up moments that we hold on to. We can close our eyes and be in so many places right now—recall the air, the sounds, the sun, the scenery—whether it's Hawaii, France, the Bahamas, Jamaica, Mexico, Italy, Costa Rica, Puerto Rico, New York, fifteen different cities on tour, or Turks and Caicos. We remember how it all felt because we were able to be fully present with ourselves and each other while we were there. Even if we were busy, we always made time to soak in everything around us. Sometimes the small moments when you pause and relax become the biggest moments.

SPIRITUAL GUIDE
to Relax

KARENA Along with our workout and meditation, we love to start each day with a few minutes of reading. Reading relaxes us and feeds our minds and souls. Books are the perfect way to discover a new perspective, feel inspired and enlightened, and spark creativity and spirituality. It's so important to us to continually challenge ourselves, discover new things, and never stop learning. And rereading a favorite book is one of the best resets we know—you're going back to the beginning of something you already know, yet you discover something new and valuable every time.

Read while you run! Well . . . not really, but hear us out. If you get lost in a book but you want to head out for a jog or need to spend a lot of time driving, try the audiobook version of it. Audiobooks will keep you company and make the time fly by!

We also love to reread passages from our favorite books—and we hope this book will be one you return to whenever you're looking for motivation. I love spiritual reads and memoirs, while Katrina picks up inspiring books on leadership, business, and health science. These motivate each of us in different ways. Here are some books we recommend:

Katrina's Favorite Books

Leaders Eat Last by Simon Sinek: This is one of those books I always come back to. No matter where you are in your career and your life, I recommend reading books on leadership. They will motivate you to take on leadership roles in all aspects of your life, whether at work

What Relaxes Me

I feel like I have the relaxation thing down. I love to unwind with a good book and be close to nature. That could mean sitting on my porch or sitting by a window. I make sure to take in my surroundings . . . the ocean breeze or the breathtaking mountains. Give me a pool float, a glass of white wine, and a book on a Saturday—it's on.

Karena

What Relaxes Me

I'm the most relaxed when I'm near water. I grew up going to Cape Cod and Lake Winnipesaukee in New Hampshire, so whenever I'm on a boat, on the beach, or by a lake, I feel relaxed and at peace. There's something about the tranquil sound of water hitting rocks, the shore, or a dock. It's also when I love to journal and write reflections, affirmations, and intentions—these are the moments when my mind is the clearest. Oh yes, and in Karena's pool, floating around with her.

Katrina

or among your friends planning trips and get-togethers. Anyone and everyone can be a leader—gain the confidence to step into the role and own it!

What Successful People Know About Leadership by John C. Maxwell: Another one on leadership. This book answers some really important questions, like "How do I become a leader if I'm more junior in my company?" and "How do I balance leading others and creating myself?"

relax

The Productivity Project by Chris Bailey: Managing our time can be a challenge because we're all constantly trying to find the balance between our careers and our families while also prioritizing ourselves. This book has some really helpful and surprising advice for upping your productivity and making the most of your time.

The Little Book of Friendship by Tiddy Rowan: Like we said before, it takes being a good friend to have good friends. It's so important to make time for others, to listen to them and be there for them, and in turn, you'll have really strong female relationships in your life.

The Universe Has Your Back by Gabrielle Bernstein: I love and adore Gabby. She has a fun way of making connecting with your spiritual side and the universe approachable for everyone. She's lighthearted and fun loving, and has had incredible experiences that led her to where she is. All of her books are so insightful. In *The Universe Has Your Back*, she shows that even the toughest times in your life are new beginnings for beautiful experiences, and she reminds you to trust your intuition. As soon as you open your eyes, you see why your life is unfolding the way it is, and that it's all leading you to the beautiful path you're on. She challenges you to shift your thinking from negative to positive and encourages you to never stop evolving.

Anything about exercise science! I love reading about the body, anatomy and physiology, nutrition science, and sports and wellness. It's what I loved most about college, and it's still super relaxing to me to read about the body and how it works. With new science always coming out, it helps me apply it to our programs at Tone It Up!

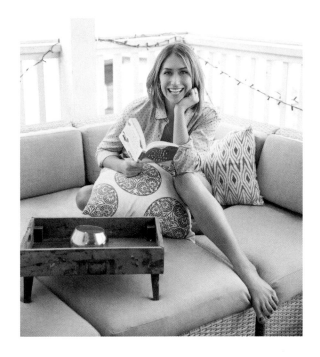

Karena's Favorite Books

A Return to Love and *A Year of Miracles: Daily Devotions and Reflections* by Marianne Williamson: She is one of the best-known motivational speakers and writers in the world, and she is just so smart, positive, and encouraging that reading anything by her instantly makes me feel centered and motivated.

Loyalty to Your Soul: The Heart of Spiritual Psychology by H. Ronald Hulnick and Mary R. Hulnick: A friend and mentor of mine suggested this book to me. I love how it explores both psychology and spirituality. It's fascinating!

relax

Four Agreements by Don Miguel Ruiz and Janet Mills: This book teaches you four daily practices to embrace love and feel like your happiest self. Trust me, this is a must read! I gave Kat a copy for her birthday this year, and I keep a copy by my couch to remind me daily that I am living by these agreements with myself: (1) Be impeccable with your word, (2) Don't take anything personally, (3) Don't make assumptions, and (4) Always do your best.

A New Earth by Eckhart Tolle: Tolle is a wonderful teacher, especially with lessons about how to live without ego and how to stop listening to that "voice in your head." By the end of the book, you will find yourself in a state of knowing how to truly live in the present. I love this quote: "Sometimes letting things go is an act of far greater power than defending or hanging on."

Tuesdays with Morrie by Mitch Albom: This may be my all-time favorite book. I've given it to so many friends as a present (including Kat!). It's a story of a man who visits his old professor Morrie, who has ALS, every Tuesday. Each time they meet, Morrie talks about a different subject on "The Meaning of Life." One of my favorite quotes to live by is "The most important thing in life is to learn how to give out love, and to let it come in."

Heal Your Body and *You Can Heal Your Life* by Louise Hay: Hay is a master of using affirmations to help you better understand and utilize the connections between your health and your emotions. Her message is so powerful.

Getting There by Gillian Segal: This is the ideal book to pick up for a quick read to get motivated. Thirty leaders share their paths to success and the hurdles they overcame to get there. I loved reading lessons from people like Jillian Michaels, Frank Gehry, Rachel Zoe, and Sara Blakely.

If you have a bit more time in the morning, delving into these memoirs will engage your emotions in the most profound way:

The Year of Magical Thinking by Joan Didion: This is one of the most moving memoirs ever written. Didion chronicles the year after her husband's sudden death from a heart attack, when they had just returned from the hospital where their only child lay in a coma. It is an incredible meditation on how to find motivation and meaning when enduring unfathomable grief.

The Glass Castle by Jeannette Walls: Walls tells the story of growing up with her unconventional and flawed family and yet carving out a successful life for herself on her own terms. It's such a moving story of self-determination, unconditional love for your family, and belief in yourself.

Love Warrior by Glennon Doyle Melton: In this powerful story, Melton shares a raw look into her life as she learns how to truly love herself after her troubled teen years and difficult marriage. It's an inspiring story of true spiritual development. In one of my favorite sections, she explains what "sexy" means to her, and this really resonated with me: "I think sexy is a grown-up word to describe a person who's confident that she is already exactly who she was made to be. A sexy woman knows herself and she likes the way she looks, thinks, and feels." This is *you*!

WORKOUT GUIDE
to Relax

If you need to unwind and release, head to a yoga class or go through a few stretches and yoga flows like this one. It's amazing what focusing on your breath can do for you, and it puts you in a calm, relaxed state. Do one or as many as you like throughout the day.

Yoga Flow to Strengthen, Focus, and Relax

With this vinyasa series, repeat the set of poses *three times* on each side:

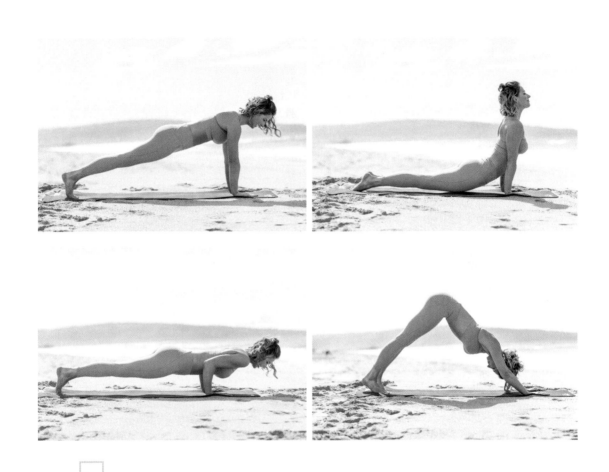

1

Plank to Chaturanga to Up Dog to Down Dog.

relax

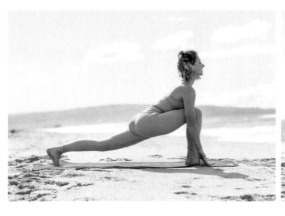

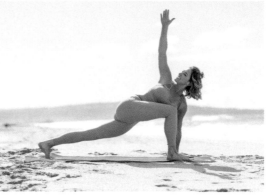

2 Step your right foot up into a low lunge, plant your left hand on the mat, and reach your right arm up to the sky for a twist.

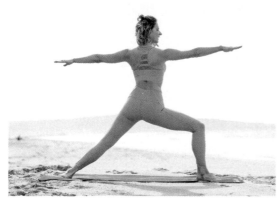

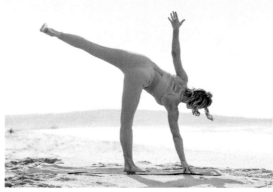

3 Lower your right hand as you plant your back heel, and open into Warrior Two.

4 Shift your weight forward into Half Moon.

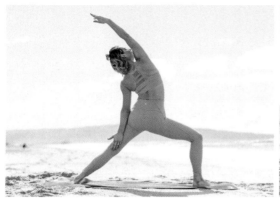

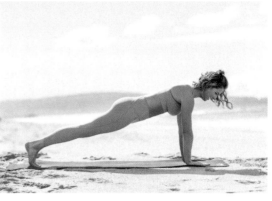

5 *Step back into Reverse Warrior.*

6 *Windmill down into Plank. Return to step 1 and repeat the series on the other side.*

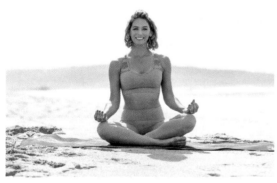

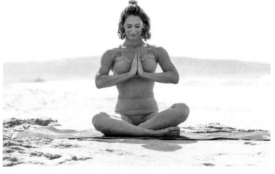

7 *Repeat the series on both sides three times, return to Down Dog, then take a seat.*

8 *Stay seated or lie on your back for 5 to 7 minutes of Savasana and meditation.*

relax

HOW TO RELEASE STRESS

Stress happens to all of us at times, and it's completely okay! These are our favorite healthy ways to de-stress:

Let it go! Letting it all out by confiding in your trusted girls who always have your back is incredibly therapeutic. When you're feeling stressed, don't keep those feelings bottled up. It's so much healthier to tell someone how you feel. Just call her up and say, "Can I vent for just a second?" We always call each other when we need to talk through something.

Stroll away the stress. If you're having a stressful day at work, take a ten-minute stroll on your next break. Exercise releases those feel-good endorphins, which can combat stress. And if you can get out in nature, even better.

Namaste. Research has linked yoga to decreased stress levels. A hot yoga class always gives us relaxed, happy vibes! Yoga will give you strength and flexibility and will improve your breathing while reducing stress.

Soothing soundtracks. Music has some powerful effects on the mind and body. Tunes with a strong beat can get you up and moving your booty (and you know exercise boosts endorphins), plus soothing sounds will calm you. Some of our favorites are listening to meditation or yoga-vibe stations on Spotify or Pandora. (Again, see our "Balanced and Beautiful" playlists on Spotify at Tone It Up.)

Make 'em laugh. Laughter really is the best medicine—the act of laughing releases endorphins. Invite your girls over for a movie night. We love *The Holiday* and *It's Complicated.*

RECIPE GUIDE
to Relax

Cooking can be an incredibly relaxing and calming thing to do, especially when you're making a recipe you love!

TONE IT UP PANCAKES

Serves 2

1 banana

1 tablespoon unsweetened almond milk

½ cup egg whites, lightly whisked

2 scoops Tone It Up Protein

1 teaspoon ground cinnamon

2 to 3 tablespoons fresh pitaya juice (to make it pink!)

Coconut oil spray

Fresh fruit, honey, or maple syrup (optional)

In a bowl, mash the banana with the almond milk. Gradually stir in the egg whites, Tone It Up Protein, cinnamon, and pitaya juice until the batter is well combined.

Coat a skillet with coconut oil spray and set it over medium-low heat. When the skillet is warm, pour in the batter evenly, shaping two pancakes, or cook one at a time if you prefer. Cook the pancakes 3 to 5 minutes on each side, or until both sides are golden brown and the pancakes are fully cooked.

Serve the pancakes topped with fresh fruit, if you like, and/or drizzled with honey or maple syrup.

relax

PINK CHOCOLATE DONUTS

Makes 10 (1 donut per serving)

½ cup chocolate Tone It Up Protein

½ cup almond meal

½ teaspoon baking soda

½ teaspoon baking powder

¼ cup unsweetened cocoa powder

¼ cup maple syrup

2 tablespoons coconut oil, melted

¼ cup egg whites, lightly whisked

¼ cup unsweetened almond milk

¼ cup Greek-style or almond yogurt

¼ cup dark chocolate chips (optional)

Coconut oil spray

FOR THE FROSTING

Coconut yogurt

Raspberries, crushed

FOR THE TOPPING (OPTIONAL)

Pink sprinkles

Preheat the oven to 350°F.

In a bowl, combine the Tone It Up Protein, almond meal, baking soda, baking powder, and cocoa powder.

Stir in the maple syrup, melted coconut oil, egg whites, almond milk, and yogurt, as well as the chocolate chips if you wish, combining everything well.

Coat a donut pan with the coconut oil spray and scoop the donut batter into it to make 10 donuts.

Bake the donuts for 15 minutes, or until a toothpick comes out clean. Let the donuts cool for a few minutes before frosting.

For the frosting, mix coconut yogurt with crushed raspberries.

Top the donuts with the frosting and pink sprinkles, if desired.

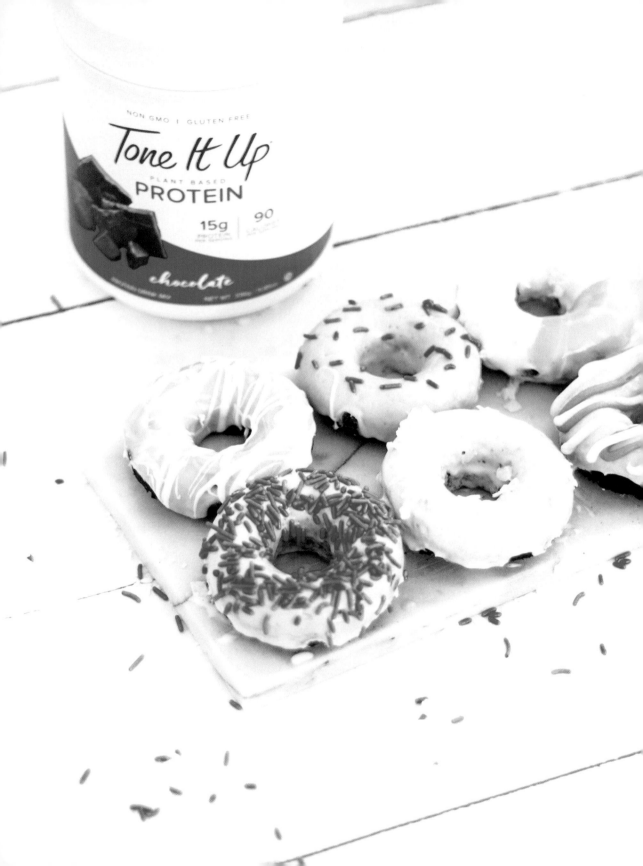

CHOCOLATE PEANUT BUTTER SMOOTHIE *of* YOUR DREAMS

Serves 1

**FOR THE
PEANUT BUTTER LAYER**

½ cup unsweetened
almond milk

½ frozen banana

1 tablespoon peanut butter

**FOR THE
CHOCOLATE LAYER**

½ cup unsweetened
almond milk

1 scoop chocolate Tone It Up
Protein

¼ cup chopped frozen
cauliflower

1 teaspoon unsweetened
cocoa powder

In a high-speed blender, blend all the ingredients of the peanut butter layer until the mixture is smooth. Pour it into a serving glass, saving a little bit to top the smoothie.

Next, blend all the ingredients of the chocolate layer until the mixture is smooth. Pour that on top of the peanut butter layer.

Drizzle over the top the last bit of the peanut butter mixture. You can also drizzle on melted dark chocolate if you're feelin' like more chocolate.

POP IT LIKE IT'S HOT POPCORN

Serves 2

½ cup popcorn kernels

1 tablespoon coconut oil

2 teaspoons sea salt

In a saucepan set over medium-high heat, warm a couple of popcorn kernels with the coconut oil. Put a lid on the saucepan and wait for the initial kernels to pop. This lets you know the heat is just right. When the pan is hot enough, add the remaining kernels and replace the lid on the pan.

Carefully shake the saucepan as the kernels pop. When they are all popped, transfer the popcorn to a bowl and toss it with the salt.

Add any of the following extra flavor options that you and your friends might like! (See photo on page 219.)

CINNAMON SUGAR

1 teaspoon ground cinnamon

1 tablespoon coconut sugar

LEMON CHIVE

2 tablespoons fresh lemon zest

½ cup chopped fresh chives

NACHO FAVORITE

1 tablespoon nutritional yeast

¼ teaspoon ground cayenne

HONEY NUT

2 tablespoons almond butter

2 tablespoons honey (soften it in a microwave first)

CHOCOLATE TRAIL MIX

2 tablespoons dark chocolate chips

2 tablespoons crushed pistachios

2 tablespoons dried cranberries or raisins

relax

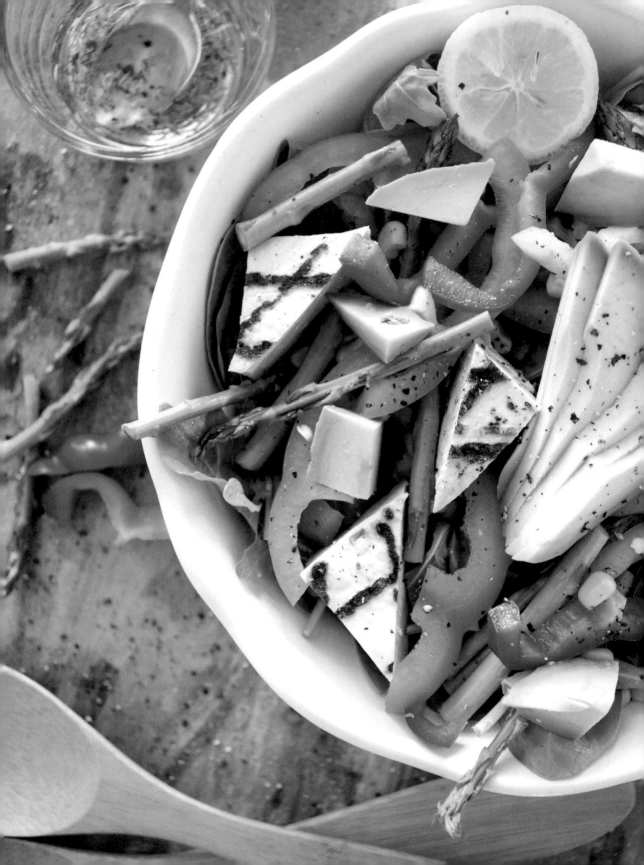

SUMMER SALAD *with* LEMON DIJON DRESSING

Serves 1

You should have enough leftover Lemon Dijon Dressing from Day 1 for this recipe too.

2 cups chopped fresh spinach

¼ cup chopped asparagus

½ cup chopped red and orange bell pepper

2 tablespoons fresh corn kernels

2 tablespoons chopped fresh basil leaves

¼ avocado, peeled, pitted, and diced

4 ounces grilled tofu, chicken, or fish

Lemon Dijon Dressing (page 13)

In a bowl, toss together all the ingredients until everything is well coated with the dressing, then serve.

relax

ZUCCHINI BIKINI PASTA
with CHICKEN MEATBALLS

Serves 3

For this recipe, you can either employ a spiralizer tool or buy spiralized zucchini noodles—your choice. For a TIU-approved marinara sauce, look for a sauce that has a short ingredient list and that's low in sodium.

1 pound ground chicken

1 teaspoon dried basil

1 teaspoon ground garlic

1/2 teaspoon salt

1 1/2 teaspoons olive oil, divided

6 large zucchini, spiralized, or 16 ounces prepackaged zucchini noodles

TIU-approved marinara sauce

Preheat the oven to 350°F.

In a bowl, combine the ground chicken with the basil, garlic, and salt. Roll the ground chicken mixture into small meatballs. Place the meatballs on a parchment paper–lined baking sheet and drizzle them with 1 teaspoon of the olive oil.

Bake the meatballs for 20 to 30 minutes, or until the meatballs are cooked through.

Heat the remaining 1/2 teaspoon olive oil in a pan set over medium-low heat, then add the zucchini noodles, sautéing them just long enough to warm them, about 3 to 5 minutes.

Meanwhile, warm the marinara sauce in a small pot over medium heat.

Serve the chicken meatballs over the zucchini noodles with 1/4 cup of the marinara sauce per serving. Save any extra in the fridge for lunch the next day!

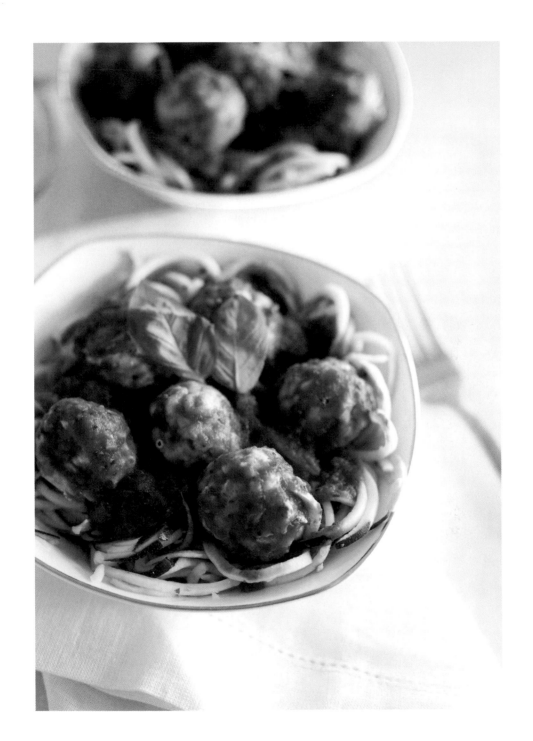

SLIM-DOWN BURGERS

Serves 2

This healthy burger is great paired with grilled asparagus and lemon.

½ pound lean ground turkey

¼ cup canned chickpeas, drained and rinsed

¼ cup egg whites

½ teaspoon garlic powder

Pinch of salt and pepper

4 portobello mushroom caps, stemmed

Any of your favorite burger toppings (we love sliced avocado, leafy greens, sliced red onion, ketchup, and mustard)

Preheat a grill. If you don't have a grill, you can cook these in a skillet set over medium heat.

In a bowl, combine the ground turkey, chickpeas, egg whites, garlic powder, salt, and pepper, stirring until the mixture is uniform in consistency, then form it into 2 patties.

Put both patties on the grill or in the preheated skillet. Cook them on each side for about 5 to 7 minutes, depending on how thick the patties are. If you're using a skillet, cook them covered for about 7 minutes on each side.

Create a burger "bun" with the mushroom caps. When the burger patties are cooked through, slide each one onto a mushroom cap, add your favorite burger toppings, then set another mushroom cap on top.

SLIMMING CAULIFLOWER PIZZA

Serves 6

This pizza is made with a cauliflower pizza crust, which you can find in the frozen foods aisle of many grocery stores, or you can be adventurous and make your own. You can also top this pizza with any other veggies you prefer. For a TIU-approved marinara sauce, look for a sauce that has a short ingredient list and that's low in sodium.

1 pre-made medium-size cauliflower pizza crust

¼ to ½ cup TIU-approved marinara sauce

Your favorite sliced veggies (we love onions, tomatoes, green peppers, and olives)

Dairy-free cheese (we love almond- or cashew-based ones)

Preheat the oven to 375°F.

Place the cauliflower pizza crust on a baking sheet lined with parchment paper.

Smooth marinara sauce over the crust, and dot it with veggies of your choice. Bake it for 10 to 15 minutes.

Pull the pizza out of the oven and top it with the dairy-free cheese, then bake it for 2 more minutes.

Allow the pizza to cool for 5 minutes before cutting and serving.

relax

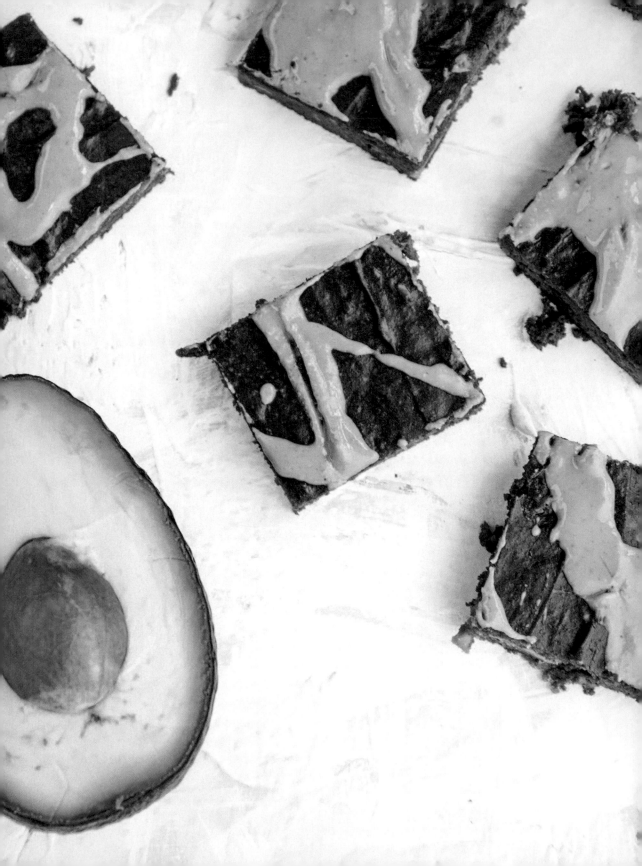

AVOCADO PEANUT BUTTER BROWNIES

Makes 9

2 avocados, peeled and pitted

2 eggs, lightly whisked

2 tablespoons coconut oil, melted

1/2 cup maple syrup

1 teaspoon vanilla extract

1/4 cup vanilla Tone It Up Protein

1/2 cup oat flour or almond flour

1/4 cup unsweetened cocoa powder

1/2 teaspoon baking powder

1/4 teaspoon sea salt

2 tablespoons peanut butter

Coconut oil spray

Preheat the oven to 350°F.

In a bowl, mash the avocado flesh, then combine it thoroughly with the eggs, melted coconut oil, maple syrup, and vanilla extract. Set the mixture aside.

In a separate bowl, combine the Tone It Up Protein, oat or almond flour, cocoa powder, baking powder, and sea salt.

Stir the wet ingredients into the dry ingredients along with the peanut butter, incorporating everything thoroughly.

Coat a 9 × 13-inch baking dish with coconut oil spray, then press the batter into the dish.

Bake the brownies for 30 minutes, or until an inserted toothpick comes out clean. Let the brownies cool for 20 minutes, then refrigerate them until you are ready to eat them. At that time, cut the mixture into 9 brownies.

relax

EAT UP
TO WIND DOWN

These foods and sips will help you get the amazing night's rest you deserve!

- Look for foods high in **tryptophan**, an amino acid that helps with the production of melatonin, the hormone that regulates your sleep–wake cycle. Go for tart cherries or unsweetened cherry juice, goji berries, almonds and other nuts, turkey and chicken, tofu, milk, lentils, and eggs.

- **Magnesium** also helps kick melatonin production into high gear. Some of the best sources are pistachios, walnuts, Greek-style yogurt, bananas, leafy greens, and black beans.

- **Tea**, please! Anything hot will be super relaxing, as long as it doesn't have caffeine. Certain teas, like chamomile, are known to help you relax and fall asleep. Ginger is also awesome, because it is very warming and aids in digestion. Passionflower tea is often used for calming anxiety, so sip away if you want some extra soothing.

LOVE TO COOK,
COOK TO LOVE

One of the best date nights is listening to music over a glass of red wine and whipping together a recipe from the Tone It Up Nutrition Plan.

Here's our guide to unwinding in the kitchen with your loved ones:

- Get your grill on! Bobby and Brian love to grill. They'll usually grill a lean protein (fish, chicken, or turkey burgers) and then tons of veggies, like asparagus, zucchini, onions, or cauliflower. Wrap some brussels sprouts in tin foil with seasoning and add it to the grill too. They come out perfect. We add a big salad, and dinner is ready!

- No grill? Our go-to dinner is cooking lean turkey in a large saucepot. We put a pound of ground turkey in the pot with 1/2 cup vegetable broth. We break up the turkey, cover the pot, and let it cook over low heat. Then we add tons of vegetables, a little bit of marinara sauce, and spices. It's so simple, and it tastes amazing!

- Make breakfast for two. We love to whip up protein pancakes or waffles on Sunday mornings (see Tone It Up Pancakes, page 201). Get a heart-shaped waffle iron and use the pancake batter for waffles instead. Try making someone heart-shaped waffles without them breaking into a huge smile!

relax

GIRLFRIEND GUIDE
to Relax

Relax with a Girls' Night In!

KATRINA Okay, picture this: you, your besties, dinner's cookin', music is on, and your favorite lineup of rom-coms is ready for you with your favorite flavored popcorn. Sometimes an intimate girls' night in is exactly what we need rather than hitting the town. Don't get us wrong. We love a night out and exploring new places, but sometimes being home with our girlfriends is just what the mind and body ordered!

Plus, yoga pants, sweater socks, and scrunchies are totally acceptable.

We put together a guide to make everything fabulous—from the menu to the personal DIY touches—so you can enjoy yourself and focus on connecting with your girls.

- Group text! Send out a text to your girls and ask them which day works for everyone. Depending on how many girls, you may need to plan a couple of weeks in advance to get everyone together.

- Make it lean, green, 'n' clean—our go-to guidelines on the Tone It Up Nutrition Plan. You want it to be as simple as possible so you don't have to spend hours cooking and can spend more time with your girls. We like the easy TIU Tray Bake (page 70), made with lean protein and lots of veggies, or a big pot of chili paired with a superfood salad. And there's always Taco Tuesdays (check out recipes on pages 157–62).

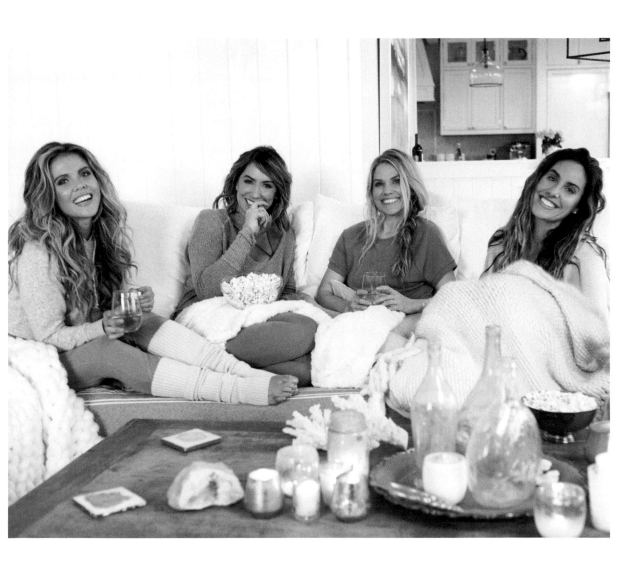

- You can also make your dinner a potluck. Your friends will be happy to bring something, especially a dish they love. Ask your girls to whip up a different appetizer, side, or dessert.

- Wine and dine! Pick up red, white, and some kombucha. Special celebration? Grab some champagne. To make things cute and personalized, write everyone's names on their glasses with a glass pen. This way no one loses track of their champs too!

- Make flower favors! As you know, I love fresh flowers. Before your girls' night, pick up a bunch of fresh flowers and mason jars. Paint the bottoms of the mason jars with spray paint for an ombré-style vase. Make the arrangements short so everyone can see each other at the table. At the end of the night, everyone gets to go home with a pretty party favor for their kitchen!

- Shake it like a Polaroid picture! One of our favorite cameras to have lying around is a Polaroid camera. We've captured some of our favorite moments on these. I created a whole album for Karena after her bachelorette weekend. Polaroid pictures also look gorgeous strung along twine in your dining room.

- End on a sweet note with a light, simple dessert. We love coconut yogurt with some fresh fruit and a little honey drizzle. Also check out the delicious dessert recipes throughout the book.

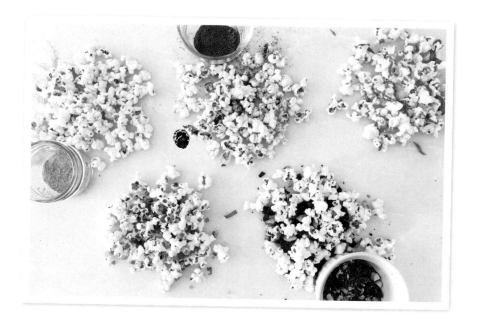

Groovy Movie Night

There are three steps to having the best movie night ever:

1. Make it comfy—gather every pillow in the house and make a huge room with pillows and blankets.

2. Set the scene—light candles and dim the lights.

3. Make popcorn!

Never have I watched *Clueless, Romeo and Juliet, Grease, Pretty Woman,* or *The Breakfast Club* without eating a bowl of popcorn. Our delicious flavoring choices for it add a fun twist to the night (page 205)!

relax

BEAUTY TIPS
to Relax

- Let your hair dry naturally or just weave it in a relaxed braid.

- Wear light makeup or go "naked" for the day to let your skin breathe.

- Take a lavender bath with Epsom salt.

- Dim the lights.

- Light candles.

- Take a mud bath.

- Go to a day spa.

- Have a massage or a facial.

- Wear loose-fitting clothing.

You're beautiful in sweatpants, fuzzy socks, no bra, and a scrunchie! Need we say more?

CONNECT WITH THE TONE IT UP COMMUNITY
to Relax

There's something about connecting with other women who are going through the same thing as you or who can just listen. It helps you relax and know that you're not alone and we're all in this together.

Stories from Community Members

Jasmine

Jasmine @jasmine_tiu

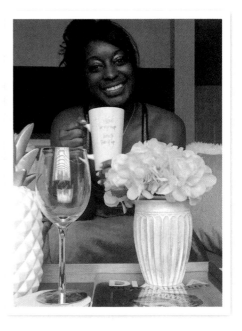

"One of my favorite things to do to relax and show my body love is taking a bath with a glass of wine, jazz music in the background, and of course candles! The more the merrier! It opens the mind, creates great energy, and makes you feel so empowered. With all of the stress that gets thrown at us every day, you *must* take some time for you and unwind, time to just let go of it all."

relax

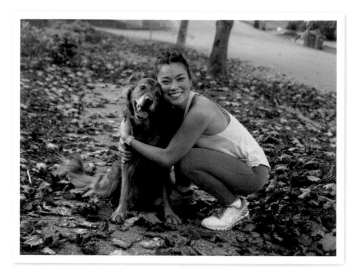

katrina and her dog

Katrina @katrina_tiu

"My life is go, go, go a lot of the time. When I get a chance to relax I need to do it completely. It might sound strange, but one of the ways I like to relax is by running outside. I love to run when I've had a stressful day, even if it's for only a mile or three. I run with my dog, Bosley, which makes him extremely happy—which in turn makes me feel even better. I stretch and pet Bosley to slow things down after our run, which creates a soothing and relaxing vibe after such an invigorating experience. Sometimes you need to get out any aggression or pent-up energy to relax your body. Think of it as priming your body for relaxation."

Stephanie

Stephanie @stephy_fitwhnp

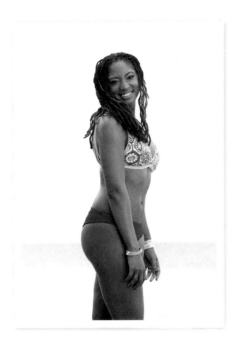

"To me, meditation means to quiet your mind and focus on the present moment, emotions, and feelings right in front of you. To be fully present with yourself in that moment. My favorite form of meditation is guided imagery, or visualization, meditation—imagining all the positive or relaxing things I need to see in that moment to help me manifest what it is that I want. By visualizing positive images, it helps me to relax and feel comforted that all will be okay."

relax

ACTION GUIDE
to Relax

When we think of relaxation, we think of winding down and enjoying being present and stress-free. With the constant hustle and bustle, it can be a challenge to take time for ourselves and kick back. Here are a few ways we ensure that we're in a state of relaxation and peace.

- Get your yoga on, anytime! Regular exercise not only gives you more energy during the day, but it helps you sleep better at night too. With the Studio Tone It Up app, you can take classes every hour on the hour from anywhere. It makes it so easy to get your workout in at any time and connect with others in the community from around the world.

- Eat early. Our bodies get going with digestion, so eating late can leave you tossing and turning. Studies have also shown that if you go for a fifteen-minute walk after dinner it helps with digestion. So after finishing up your meal, take a stroll around your neighborhood. Use this time to listen to a podcast or music, call a friend to check in, or just be mindful of how nice it is to be outside. Eating your dinner earlier also gives you more time to wind down and set your intentions for tomorrow.

- Sometimes an intense workout gets us super wired, and it can keep us up later at night. If you didn't have the chance to work out earlier in your day, choose a routine in Studio Tone It Up

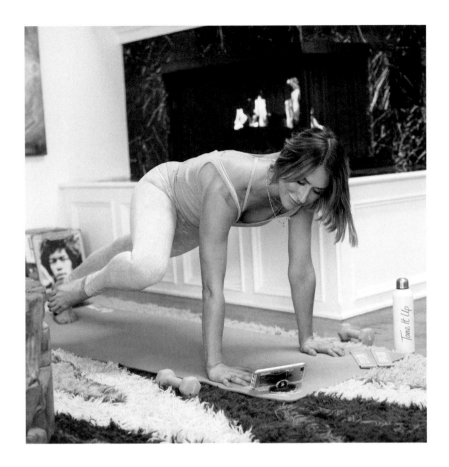

that is better for the evening, like yoga sculpt, restorative yoga, toning, or stretching.

- Create your own special wind-down routine before bed. We recommend putting the phone away, lighting a candle, putting your feet up, and journaling. Taking a few moments for yourself is the best way you can relax after a long day.

relax

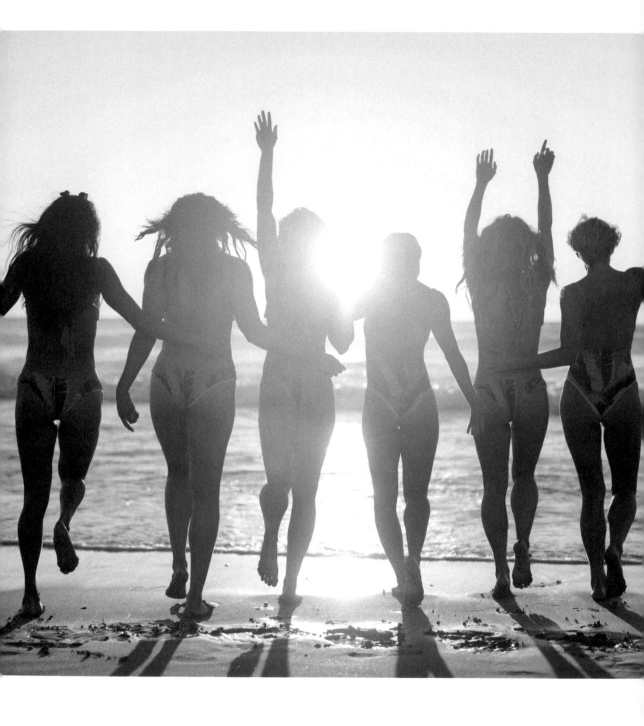

Sunsets to Relax

Sunsets have been a huge part of our life together and Tone It Up—living by the beach and walking together, visualizing building a community while the sun goes down, going for sunset runs, watching sunsets from our Tone It Up HQ, ending a long day of filming a HIIT or yoga workout at sunset, or watching the sun go down on other beaches around the world. The sun setting is a representation of an ending and a new beginning. There's something really beautiful about seeing the sun dip down and being fully present with it. Feeling connected and reflecting on the significance and magnitude is so important.

Here are some tips on how to make sure you always see that sunset:

- Drop everything! Even when we're still at the office, we leave our computers, put down our phones, and watch the sun go down. If you're at home and super busy, just remind yourself to pause and be present before the day ends. It helps to put your phone aside—unless of course you're snapping a pic for Instagram!

- Plan a Happy Hour. Go out and watch the sun set over the mountains with a bunch of healthy apps and a glass of wine. You can also pack a bag for a sunset picnic. We try to do this once a month with friends and family to make it special.

- Make it a tradition. It's important to have "your thing"—your time to connect with yourself and the day. Now is the best time to start rituals and make little things just something that you do every day!

relax

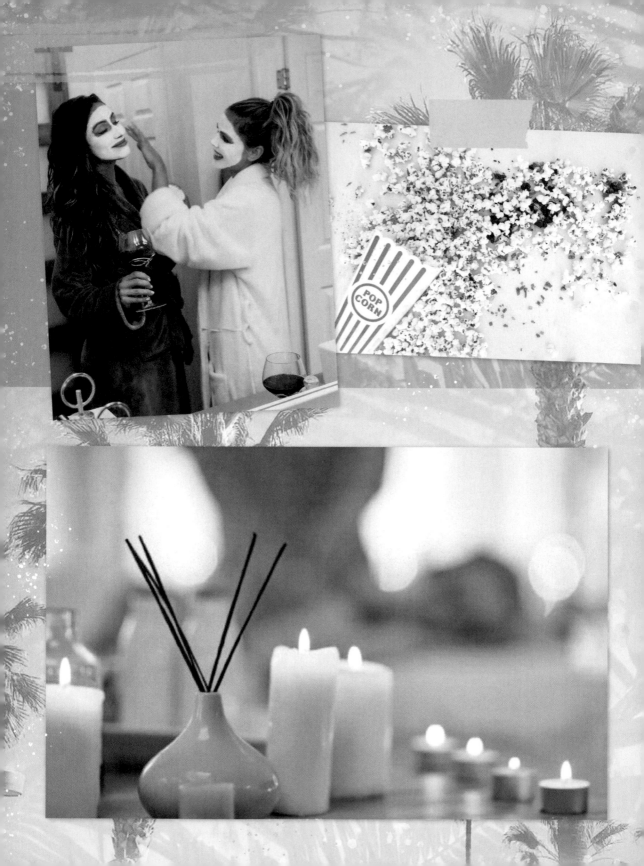

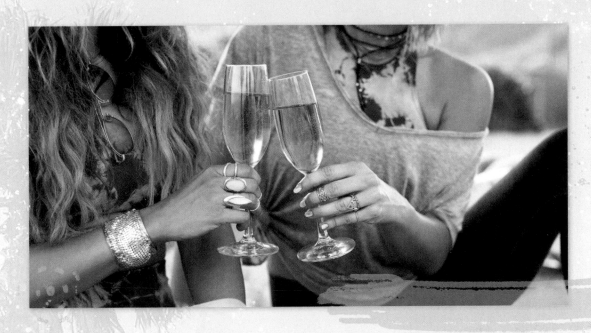

Vision Board to Relax

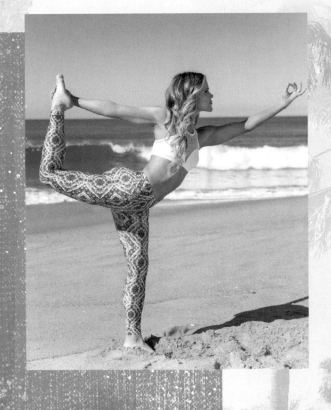

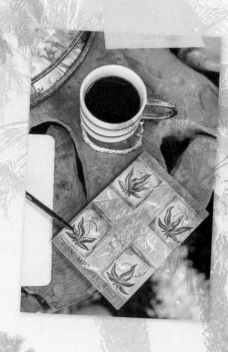

REFLECT
to Relax

I feel most relaxed when I

_____

My favorite relaxing food or drink is

_____

If relaxation had a sound, it would be

_____

Something I would love to do that I know will be relaxing is

_____

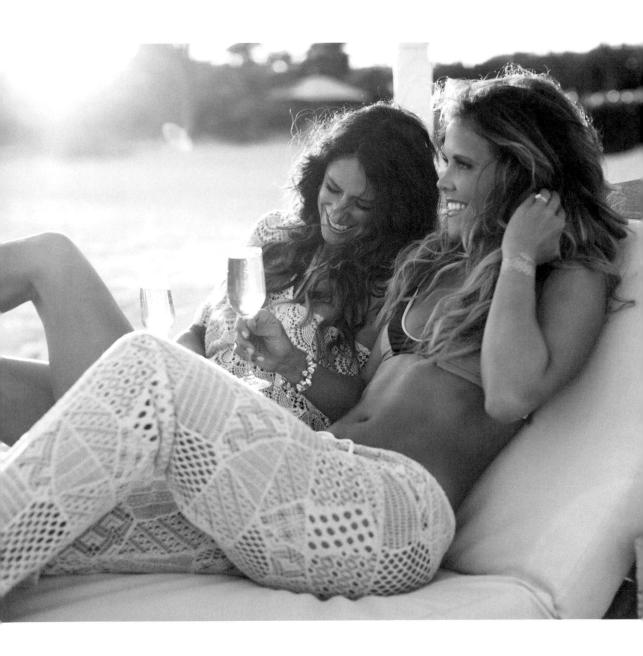

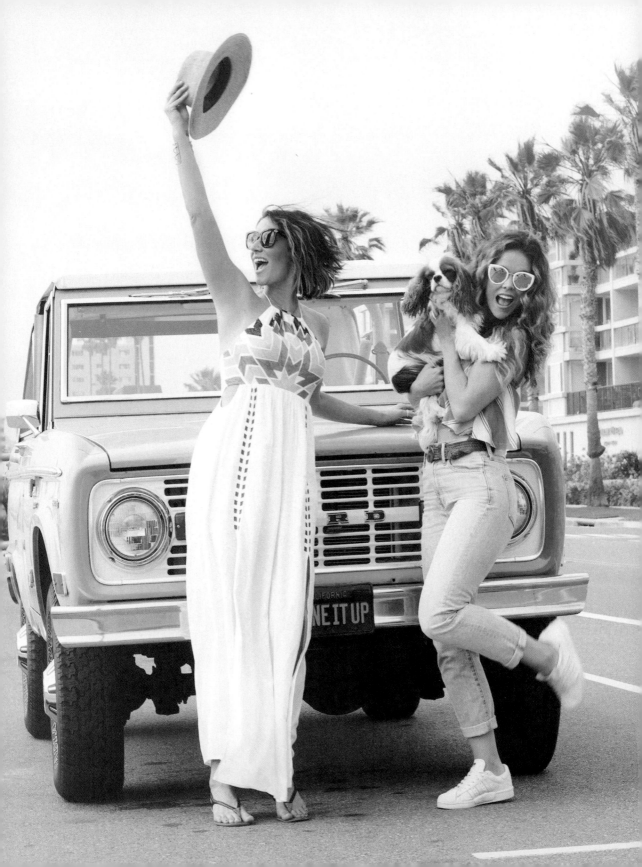

You're Balanced and Beautiful

As we come to the end of this book, remember it's just the beginning of your journey—it's time to create your story. You've looked inward in your pursuit of balance and beauty, and now you have the tools, the ideas, the positive vibes, and a community filled with supportive women to help you live your best life.

We want to take a moment to say how proud we are of you. It takes courage to pause and make time for *you*. Like a best girlfriend, this book and the Tone It Up community will always be here for you. Whenever you need us, you know where to turn. Whenever you have a success to be celebrated, share it with us. Whenever you need a boost, we're here to lift you up. We're here every day—every step of the way.

Whether you're looking to feel *refreshed, motivated, inspired, energized,* or *relaxed,* come back to these pages. The best investment you can make is the one of self-discovery and personal growth, using your passion and love.

Lastly . . . like we said in the beginning, this balanced and beautiful life is already *yours*—you are strong, you are gorgeous, you are brilliant, you are loved, and you are enough. Here's to you and your bright future!

With so much love,

Karena and Katrina

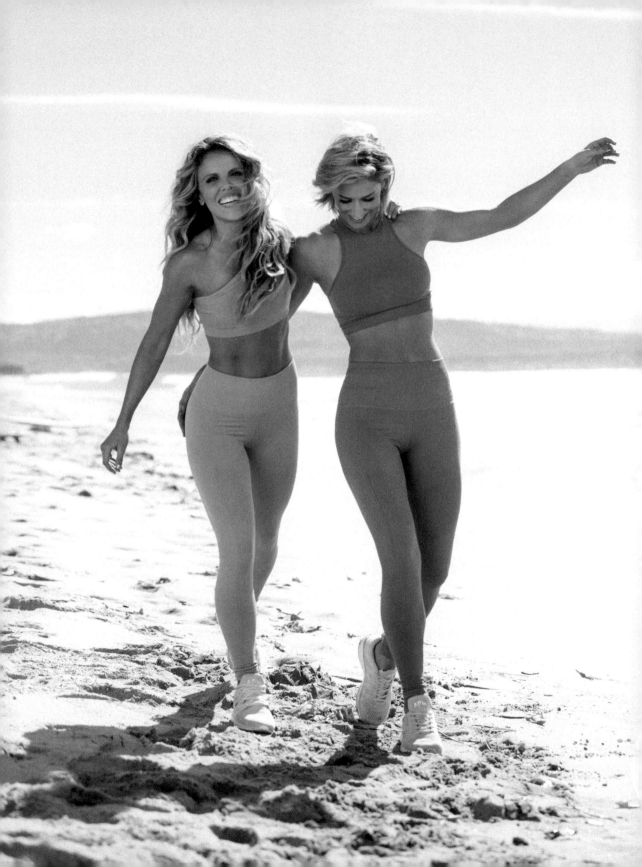

ACKNOWLEDGMENTS

We are forever grateful

for everyone who continues to support us through this beautiful journey!

Love to our families and our husbands, Bobby and Brian, who are our biggest support system through everything.

A big hug and thanks to our girlfriends who shared their unfiltered advice and tips on breakups, self-love, and keeping friendships strong. This book is filled with inspiration from all of you.

To the Tone It Up community, we are so grateful for the love and dedication you share with us and each other, every day. All of you are our motivation and strength!

Thank you to our Tone It Up team members, who pour so much love, care, and devotion into their careers at TIU HQ!

A special thanks to our agent, Eileen Cope, for always believing in our vision. And to Gideon Weil, Hilary Lawson, and Sydney Rogers at HarperCollins, for sharing our message with the world.

And a huge thanks to the rest of the remarkable team—we couldn't have done this without you: Karen Moline, Bailey Julio, Nicole Hill, Jenna Anton, Ashley Kucich, and Allie Baker! You babes rock our world.

And lastly, to our friendship and love—without each other, none of this would be possible!

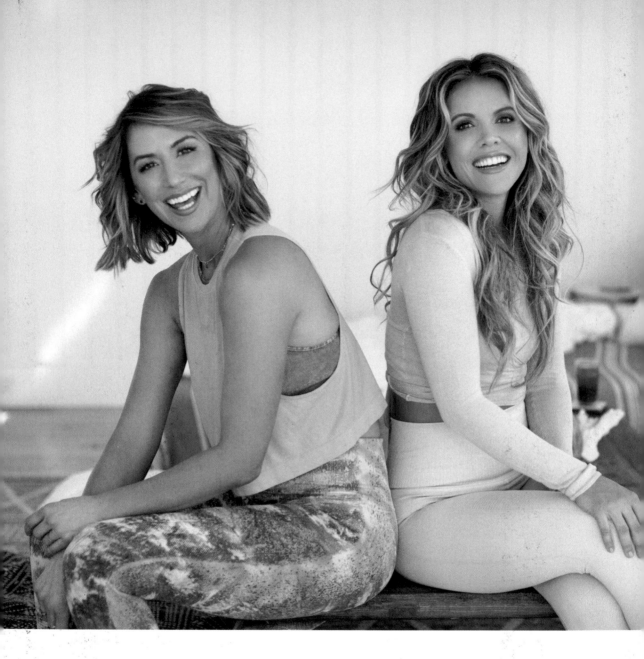

xo, K+K